Praise for Jeremy Ueno, and *Oral Fitness*

Dr. Ueno has taken care of my periodontal well-being for the past seven years, including during a time of ill health. He provided beneficial and progressive surgeries that improved my situation and restored my gums to excellent health. His caring and professional approach to providing advanced treatment is greatly appreciated. I am very happy to be his patient.

—Mirelle Nunan

Thank you Dr. Ueno and staff for a job well done on the surgery and implant you did for me. I am happy with the result. Dr. Ueno was so gentle throughout the process, and the staff was always responsive when I had questions regarding the procedure and my insurance coverage. The receptionist even helped me with the door when I was walking on crutches. All in all, I highly recommend Dr. Ueno and his staff to others requiring periodontal work; you could not find a better place.

—Avelina Simpliciano

Dr. Ueno has taken care of the periodontal health of my family for years. I've received wonderful care from him and so has my fiancé. Dr. Ueno's intervention saved my fiancé from a medical emergency that could have cost him his life. My fiancé wasn't aware of his extremely high blood pressure (high to the point of likely imminent heart attack), and once Dr. Ueno examined him and counseled him on the risk, my fiancé rushed to get emergency care. Fortunately he was treated in time and we owe it all to Dr. Ueno, who not only identified the severe risk, but explained the critical connection between gum/dental health and overall physical health, whether it is high blood pressure or A1C. Dr. Ueno has performed surgeries on both of us and we're so happy about the very successful outcomes. He handled my first implant, which I was I was very nervous about, but he made me feel so comfortable. The process went so smoothly and I feel so fortunate that we found such an amazing, gifted, and caring doctor! We highly recommend him.

—Anonymous patient

ORAL FITNESS

How Complete Health Dentistry
is *Revolutionizing America*

JEREMY K. UENO, DMD

WITH: **Charles Whitney, M.D.**

Michael L. Gelb, DDS, MS

Gina L. Pritchard, MSN, RN, CNS, ACNP, DNPc

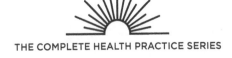

THE COMPLETE HEALTH PRACTICE SERIES

CONTENTS

CHAPTER 1

HOW MY JOURNEY BECAME A JOURNEY FOR OTHERS

We have all heard the saying "What doesn't kill you only makes you stronger." While there can be some truth to that, in my health and fitness journey, the more appropriate phrase is "The *fear* of what can kill you only makes you stronger."

During my surgical training at Columbia University, I was taught the oral-systemic connection. When I started practicing, patients would ask me about it, and I would give them basic information. I had trouble correlating it to their lives because at the time, I was young. Looking back, I realized that even though I talked about it, I did not own it because I was not personally invested. It took me becoming unhealthy and taking a journey back to health, along with the perfect storm of oral-systemic continuing education, for me to be fully invested and recommitted to implementing certain parameters in my practice. The journey has helped shape who I am and what my practice is today. Also, with the COVID-19 pandemic, it has never been more important for people to be healthy, and I am proud that my practice makes people healthier through the oral-systemic connection.

I'm a fifth-generation Japanese American. Ethnically I am Japanese, but my upbringing was more "Hawaiian style." What does that mean? Well, I am an American, and my diet was a mixture of all Asian foods; however, we still celebrated the important holidays, like New Year's, with Japanese traditions.

My parents were not overly strict. In fact, my dad always said that his parenting style was to give me enough rope to not hang myself. I was a troublemaker growing up and often found myself in the principal's office. Although I had a "rope," self-discipline was always an underlying theme in my upbringing. My grandfather was especially self-disciplined. At one point in his life, he was overweight and a smoker. Something for him had to change, and through his self-discipline as a former black belt in judo, he was able to flip the switch fairly easily. In his journey back to health, he quit smoking cold turkey and switched his diet to eating natural and healthy foods. When we would go for walks, he would pick watercress and eat it like it was the most delicious food in the world. He was even eating plain oatmeal with broccoli for his breakfast! No matter what he ate, he always made it look delicious, and it would make me want to try it, but it is hard to eat plain oatmeal and broccoli, especially as a kid. He and my dad would tell me stories about the samurai and how their discipline made them great. I did not think much of this when I was a kid, but these undertones of discipline are the main reason why I was able to be successful in my journey back to health.

I've also learned that, genetically, I am more susceptible to cancer, diabetes, and other diseases since I've lost many family members to them. Now that I have three children, I've really begun to focus on the health of my entire family. But for me alone, understanding "good health" and what worked best for me was quite a struggle. Things that worked for me in my twenties no longer worked for me in my thirties. When I hit my forties, I knew it was not going to be any easier, and thus, I had to make some drastic changes to my lifestyle.

MY OWN HEALTH YO-YO

As a youth, I spent a lot of time trying to find a balance between nutrition and exercise. I was a fat kid growing up. In middle school, I was six feet and over 190 pounds at thirteen years old. Then, in high school, my basketball coach asked that I lose some weight so I could be quicker going into my sophomore season. I began to control my caloric intake to a fault and ended up a sickly looking 158 pounds. Definitely did not help my basketball game being that thin. With protein shakes and weight lifting, I reached a healthier 170 pounds during my junior year. I really started hitting the weights in my junior to senior year and reached 212 pounds by graduation. At that point, I really focused mostly on calories and never thought about the foods I was eating. I ate a box of cereal daily along with other processed foods since they were easy calories to take in. Thankfully, my mom always cooked healthy meals, so I always had a good nutritional foundation despite my poor choices.

In college, I no longer had my mom to cook healthy meals for me. I lived in the dorms and had a microwave, small fridge, and rice cooker. I ate dorm food along with lots of Spam, burritos, and beer, and I ballooned up to over 260 pounds in my junior year at the University of California at San Diego. I was so fat that my dad didn't recognize me at the airport when he came to pick me up for Thanksgiving! He literally walked right past me. I had to make a change!

I focused solely on caloric restriction (again), much like I had in high school to drop weight for basketball. At that time, I was told that I had to eat five to six small meals a day to keep my metabolism up. Through diet and exercise, I managed to drop over forty pounds between my junior and senior year. I got to 215 pounds and was in great shape and was able to stay there through dental school and my residency. I was in my twenties, had two rounds of being overweight in high school and in college, and I did not want this to happen again. In dental school at Tufts, I worked out like a maniac, lifting weights daily, playing basketball, and running four miles during my lunch breaks. During my residency at Columbia, I kept up a similar routine, plus just living in New York City, I naturally walked a lot. I was in the best shape of my life! But I had no kids, a lot of free time to work out, and again, I was in my twenties. After I graduated from my periodontal residency at Columbia, I knew I was stepping into the real world, but that real world in my mind was only work. I did not think about how having kids, getting older, and running a business would affect my health.

In 2009, my wife, Stephani, and I moved to San Jose, California, where I grew up. We met in dental school and were both about to start our dental careers. We got married in 2012 and had our first child, Skylar, in 2013. I was working incessantly on my practice and noticed that I was starting to gain some weight despite still playing basketball. I was lifting less and drinking more because I had many social events for my business. I was starting to realize that my metabolism might be slowing down in my thirties, but I did not have the insight to look myself in the mirror and call myself a lazy slob.

Then, in 2015, while in my midthirties and just having our second child, Riley, I tore my right Achilles playing basketball. After two surgeries, I had limited mobility for over a year. I rode a scooter around the office for weeks and went home at night too exhausted to play with my kids. Even worse, I still drank a decent amount to help me unwind. Through a sedentary lifestyle, eating unhealthily, and drinking, I gained fifty pounds (again!).

Finally, after my sister-in-law expressed concern about my health, I hired a personal trainer in August 2016, which was one year after my first Achilles surgery. Her exact words were, "You are really fat, and you need to do something."

I also hired a nutritionist for meal planning. Her plan for me was really simple. Just eat natural foods. Nothing processed, nothing canned, and nothing with ingredients you cannot pronounce. Basically, anything that my grandmother could not recognize as food, don't eat it. She gave me sample meal plans, and I tried to follow them initially, but I failed. I felt that natural foods were expensive and took more time to prepare. Even though I failed in this endeavor with the nutritionist, everything she said stuck with me, and that became a critical stepping-stone in my health journey.

The father of Western medicine, Hippocrates, famously said, "Let food be thy medicine, and let medicine be thy food." As Americans, we eat the *least* amount of natural foods and are the *least* healthy country in the world! So what my nutritionist told me was known centuries before!

I continued with my trainer, Matt. I felt "in shape" because I was one of the strongest people in the gym, but I was wearing size 38 pants and XXL shirts. I remember the day when I got on the scale and it read 268.5 pounds. I was bench-pressing over 350 pounds at this time, which validated the weight gain in my mind, but it was the heaviest I had ever been in my life. That was in the summer of 2018, and I knew I had to make changes in my life because we now had three kids, and I needed to have the energy and health to not only play with them but be on this earth with them for as long as possible.

Around this time, we started to work with NextLevel Practice (NLP) as our practice consultants. I liked NLP's philosophy of connecting oral and systemic health. We have always talked about the connections of the mouth and the body to our patients, but NLP helped us convey our message in a more powerful way. Also, the more I talked about the oral-systemic connection, the more I kept thinking that I had to practice what I was preaching. That year at my physical, my cholesterol and blood lipid levels were through the roof. I was in my thirties and was put on meds! This was a low time in my life as I thought I took relatively good care of myself. It would become one of my many wake-up calls.

I started eating better after that summer and was able to drop roughly ten to fifteen pounds in the first couple of months. By the end of 2018, I was down to about 250 pounds and feeling good about myself but thought I could not lose any more no matter how hard I tried. I mean, I had woken up every morning at five-thirty for the previous two years to go work out and was still struggling with my weight. What was I doing wrong?

My life changed when my wife's cousin invited me to enter a sixty-day weight-loss challenge with about ten of his friends in January 2019. It was perfect timing for me because I was dealing with the frustrations of my weight-loss stagnation. The rules of the challenge were simple: lose the highest amount of fat percentage with a $200 buy-in for a winner-take-all $2,000 pot. Awesome! That was definitely a motivating factor. I started talking to my trainer more about nutrition, and he talked to me about intermittent fasting (IF).

He had talked to me for about a year about IF, but I always told him that it would be too hard for me to do.

The $2,000 pot inspired me to start IF, which, needless to say, required a lot of discipline. The rules of IF are very simple. Simply, do not eat for a prolonged period of time, and only eat within a certain window. The first window I tried was the traditional 16:8 method. For this, you fast for sixteen hours and then eat during an eight-hour period. I would therefore eat only between the hours of noon and 8 p.m. It was tough at first, but then I realized I was only missing breakfast. The theory behind IF is that it takes your body a tremendous amount of energy to digest the food you eat. If you limit the time that you eat, your body has a chance to repair itself while not digesting food. This includes your immune system and brain. The term is *autophagy*, and this can occur only after fourteen-plus hours of fasting. In fact, the longer you fast, the more autophagy you can achieve. Fasting also increases neurogenesis and immune system repair and increases growth hormone, just to name a few benefits. Along with that, you are creating a caloric deficit, which leads to increased weight loss.

The first week of IF, I dropped seven pounds. Surprisingly, my energy was higher, and I was feeling motivated to do more. Since my buddies and I are all in our forties, we always talk about ways to try to stay young. A few of my friends were doing keto or low-carb diets. The theory behind these diets is also relatively simple. By reducing your carbohydrate intake, your body can no longer use glycogen for fuel. Instead, your body will switch to ketones for energy, which are by-products of fat. So, if you reach "ketosis," you are literally burning fat for energy. In the keto diet, you eat a high level of fat and protein and few to no carbohydrates. Eating a bunch of bacon and butter to lose weight sounded great to me!

By reducing my carb intake, I lost over twenty pounds in the sixty-day challenge, including only two-and-a-half pounds of lean muscle mass—a significantly better ratio than everyone else in the competition. We did hydrostatic body testing at baseline and at sixty days, and most people who lost significant weight also lost significant lean muscle mass. In fact, most people were losing closer to a 50-50 fat-to-lean-muscle-mass ratio. I actually did not end up losing the most weight by percentage; however, I had the least amount of lean muscle mass lost (which I attributed to heavy weight lifting four to six days per week and a high-protein, low-carb diet), and that is what secured me the win!

> Nutrition and discipline are the keys to better oral and physical health, which then leads to better systemic health.

IF is now my lifestyle. On days that I do not work, I fast for sixteen hours and eat only during an eight-hour window, just like how I started. On days that I work, I am extremely busy, and thus, I fast for twenty-two hours and eat during a two-hour window. With my new lifestyle, I have lost over 50 pounds of fat!

IF and a low-carb diet have not only made me healthier; they have actually helped me be more productive since I am not spending time trying to figure out what to eat for two meals a day. I therefore get a lot of my work finished during "lunch." This allows me to leave the office after my last patient instead of staying another hour or more doing paperwork, which gives me more time with my family.

Why does all this talk about nutrition and discipline matter to you? Because nutrition and discipline are the keys to better oral and physical health, which then leads to better systemic health. My journey was not easy, and I stumbled multiple times in my life. As

I grew older and my circumstances changed, I needed to find new ways to motivate myself and find what worked for me. Everyone is looking for a miracle pill, but those do not exist. What we choose to put in our mouths and how we treat our bodies can be 100 percent controlled. Healthier habits in my daily life led to a healthier me. If I had not made these changes, I do not know where I would be ten-plus years down the line. My latest physical shows that I am in better health now in my forties than I ever was in my thirties. When I talk to my patients about oral-systemic health, I believe my message is clearer because I walked in the shoes of being unhealthy, and it is a place I do not want to go back to. I've realized that health is one thing we all take for granted until we lose it.

THE AIRWAY—A LIFE-CHANGING LINK

The more I learn about nutrition, the more I recognize its links to our health. For instance, I brought my entire team to the NLP Summit in 2019 in Scottsdale, Arizona. There, a medical doctor discussed the benefits of fasting and how it decreases the risk of Alzheimer's disease. On top of that, fasting, along with a low-carbohydrate diet, limits the insulin spikes that your body goes through and thus reduces your risk for diseases like diabetes. Diabetes and Alzheimer's disease are very closely related. The doctor recommended a very easy fasting protocol of a twelve-hour fast and then no caloric intake for three hours before bedtime. Awesome! I was already doing this!

He then discussed how sleep or airway (the ability for us to take in oxygen) increased the risk of Alzheimer's disease. Many people in the world suffer from obstructive sleep apnea. When you have any level of sleep apnea, you will have a difficult time getting into the deep sleep when your body recovers, called rapid eye movement

(REM). In REM sleep, your brain also recovers via the "glymphatic system," which filters toxins in the brain. If you have sleep apnea, your brain is not able to rid itself of toxins daily, leading to toxin buildup and a higher risk of Alzheimer's disease. I had a light-bulb moment as my grandmother died of complications with Alzheimer's disease, so it is a subject close to my heart.

In my quest to be healthier and breathe better, I had ear, nose, and throat (ENT) surgery to fix a deviated septum I suffered over twenty years ago from multiple sports injuries. Before the surgery, I had more than 90 percent blockage in my left nostril and did not think anything of it. Now I breathe and sleep better than anytime I can remember! I wake up refreshed every morning and feel younger because of it! Sometimes I do think: Would my life be different today if I had had the surgery done twenty years ago? Would I have been healthier? I do not want to have to ask these questions about my kids, and thus, we are addressing their airway issues now.

Another concern for people with a compromised airway is the increased risk of attention deficit disorder (ADHD). The dental and medical professions believe that a child not being able to breathe well at night contributes to ADHD. Because of this, a child may wake up hundreds of times a night and not know it. If your body is not getting the oxygen that it needs, you will become more "sympathetic" and produce epinephrine (the fight-or-flight hormone). Sympathetic activity increases heart rate and arouses the sleeper to wake up and breathe to get more oxygen. If that happens hundreds of times throughout the night, the child has a lot of stored sympathetic energy. Then that child goes to school with all of that untapped energy but also is mentally fatigued from not getting deep and restful sleep; behavioral problems often result. They are then put on medications, which worsens the problem. Instead of putting these kids on medications, we want to try to screen these kids early.

Sadly, I have had many patients referred to me to be evaluated for airway issues who are in their thirties. Incredibly, almost every one of these patients was diagnosed with ADHD as a child. Would their lives be different today if they were treated for their airway issues as kids instead of given meds?

I opened a learning center called the Practi(CE)nter to facilitate important meetings with local dentists and have had a big focus on the advances and knowledge on airway. Admittedly, it was a novel subject for me as a periodontist when I first began learning about it in 2015. But the more I've learned, the greater effect it has had on my family, friends, patients, and myself. It's been mind boggling to learn about the connections between airway issues and systemic health, including the following:

- Cardiovascular disease
- Hypertension
- Stroke
- Cancer
- Alzheimer's
- Dementia
- ADHD
- Gastroesophageal reflux disease
- Preterm, low-birth-weight babies
- Restless leg syndrome
- Bed-wetting
- Night terrors
- Autism
- Bruxism
- Temporomandibular joint disorder
- Periodontal disease
- Gum recession
- Myofascial pain

Dentists can be the first line of defense to triage and diagnose these patients—this was a call to action for me.

A TURNING-POINT DIAGNOSIS

I mentioned previously, my oral-systemic journey was kick-started in 2017 after I attended a Perio Protect meeting in Las Vegas where I saw Gary Kadi, the CEO of NLP, in tears as he talked about his autistic son. The focus of this meeting was how oral disease affected our patients' systemic diseases and how we could better educate and treat our patients. I was moved by his presentation, and little did I know how this was going to personally affect me.

That turning point came in December 2018, when my oldest son, Riley, was diagnosed with moderate functioning autism. At first we were lost and did not know what to do or who to turn to. We now embrace the challenge and, as a result, have seen a huge improvement in him as a person and in our relationship as a family. Through special education schooling; speech therapy; occupational therapy; applied behavior analysis (ABA) services; and programs such as gymnastics, swimming, and other activities, we have watched him transform—leaving "his world" to become more of a "normal kid." We have also altered his diet, as gluten-free and/or low-carb diets have been proven to help people with autism spectrum disorder.

What does an autism diagnosis have to do with the airway? A link has been made between mothers who have upper airway resistance syndrome (UARS), which is closure of the airway during sleep, and children born with autism. As previously discussed, people with airway issues have an increase in sympathetic activity when they sleep. In pregnancy, this can cause an increase in the fetal intracranial pressure, which is believed to be a factor in autism of the child.

My wife has UARS, and when all of this came together, it was life altering.

Since our son's diagnosis, I have been committed to helping everyone, especially kids, breathe better. I want to help people reach their full potential and potentially reduce the incidences of children born with autism.

As a periodontist, I can also help with another part of the airway equation, a condition known as tongue-tie, where the lingual frenulum—the band of tissue on the underside of the tongue that connects it to the floor of the mouth—is unusually short or tight. The tongue plays a huge role in the development of a child's skull. Ideally, a child's lips should be closed, their tongue should be on the roof of their mouth, and they should be breathing through their nose. The pressure from the tongue on the upper jaw causes expansion of the skeleton and opens up the airway. Tongue-ties can cause a deficient maxilla, or upper jaw, because the tongue cannot reach the maxilla. Since the roof of the mouth is the floor of the nasal passages, a deficient maxilla can mean narrower nasal sinuses, which can lead to apnea. This leads to problems like ADHD and both physical and mental developmental issues. But tongue-ties can be corrected through a fairly simple surgical procedure known as a lingual frenectomy, along with oral exercises through a myofunctional therapist. I can also recognize when a child needs orthodontics to help expand their jaws or surgery and refer them.

By identifying these issues early, I can be part of the team that helps people grow to their full potential and decrease their chances of developing neurocognitive deficiencies. In fact, we have put my autistic son through myofunctional therapy and started to do work to expand his upper jaw to help him breathe better. We literally saw changes in him instantaneously. My son could not say any words in early 2019, and just a few months later, he is singing songs and saying full sentences. In 2020, he has graduated from his ABA services and is attending a mainstream kindergarten!

Through the systems that I learned in NLP, and the education I received through institutions like Spear Education, I am helping patients better understand the oral-systemic connection. The core of our practice is always excellent dentistry, and I believe that the focus on oral-systemic disease and airway really sets our practice apart.

A DIFFERENT WAY OF LOOKING AT TREATMENT

I owed it to my patients and my team to bring oral-systemic education more aggressively into my practice. There was a lot of resistance at first; however, my team loved learning about the connections because they saw how it affected them personally. There was also resistance because we were implementing all new systems, and with new systems comes a lot of training and work. So, it took over a year to get everyone on board. But ultimately, the oral-systemic connection unified my team.

Today, we look at patients differently. For those with periodontal disease, we like to start treatment with baseline bacterial testing. With this information, we can tell patients if they have bacteria in their mouths that are more aggressive, as it places them at a higher risk for not only losing their teeth but also for worsening systemic disease. We also do a genetic test on our patients to see their susceptibility for disease and whether they are more prone to being hyperinflammatory. These tests are an additional cost, and not every patient says yes to them, but the information that we gain is invaluable in educating the patient about *their* true risk for oral and systemic disease.

We talk to patients about their sleep. Do you wake often during sleep, snore, fall asleep during the day, or feel tired? A yes to these questions can mean they have an airway issue.

We have built a team that includes orthodontists, myofunctional therapists, oral surgeons, ENTs, and other specialists. Also, to ensure we're offering patients the most up-to-date diagnosis and treatment, we have brought in the latest technologies, including lasers, scanners, digital imaging, and more.

Once we educate our patients on how their oral health relates to their systemic health, they have a whole new level of appreciation for what we can do for them. Often, a patient is referred to our office because they have gum recession or need an implant, and we see other underlying issues that may have contributed to this patient's current disease. I have had patients cry at the consultations because they were so happy that they could be helped!

Whatever the treatment, we want to be sure it is the best for each patient, which may include a referral to another provider within our network. We also want to be sure we financially fit the treatment into anyone's lifestyle, whatever their needs are, and that includes different financing options.

Unfortunately, despite our efforts, some patients do not accept treatment, and they may suffer serious consequences. Teesha is an example of a patient who was initially resistant to the idea of the oral-systemic connection, didn't like our fees, and disregarded what we said. We diagnosed her with severe periodontal disease and recommended laser gum surgery. We let her know that if she did not have any treatment performed, she was at high risk of losing her teeth and that the inflammation in her mouth could affect the rest of her body. She left our office for years, and we did not see her until she was diagnosed with uncontrolled diabetes and her medical doctor made her come back to see us. We performed an FDA–approved laser treatment called Laser-Assisted New Attachment Procedure (LANAP), and she committed to her oral health. In just a few months, her diabetes and periodontal disease were under control. She was taken off multiple medications and was able to keep all her teeth. Talking to me about her outcomes brought her to tears. In addition to better oral health, she had lost weight, was living her "best life," and was looking forward to a longer and healthier life with her newfound health.

As a referral office, we typically do not see patients again if they opt out of treatment—that is, until their problems worsen to the point of eliminating many options. When a patient returns to us some time later, they typically have worsening disease that affects them systemically. New more aggressive plans often have to be made.

IT'S ABOUT HELPING PEOPLE LIVE LONGER, HEALTHIER LIVES

Another thing that attracts people to our practice is our philanthropy. I travel to Guatemala every couple of years to treat patients in underserved areas. The group that I travel with is phenomenal, and all the doctors are great clinicians. I learn a lot by just being around the top people in their field. Also, the feeling we get of helping the underserved communities is very rewarding.

Recently, since my son's diagnosis, I have focused on autism awareness. I hosted a silent auction within my local dental community since we, as dental providers, can help with airways and hopefully reduce the prevalence of autism. We raised and donated over $7,600 for a local autism charity called Parents Helping Parents (PHP.com), which was a community that gave us guidance when we first got our son's diagnosis.

My wife and I also worked with the San Jose Sharks' minor league team, the San Jose Barracudas, to host an Autism Awareness Night at the Shark Tank in March 2020. Since many kids with autism have sensory issues, the event's lights were to be dimmed and sound reduced, and there would have been multiple autism charities on the concourse, including dental offices to help spread the word of airway issues. Unfortunately, this event was canceled due to COVID-19, but we plan to reschedule the event.

These are just a few of the ways I help others. You see, I used to think that I was "just a dentist," and I could only help people by putting implants in their mouths so that they could eat and look better. Now I realize that I have the means to help people live longer, healthier lives. For me to find my way, I had to fail in my own health.

Now let me tell you how my journey to better health has turned into a journey to better health for so many other people.

CHAPTER 2

A REVOLUTION TAKES ROOT

As I mentioned in chapter one, I really started trying to make the connection between oral and systemic health after the NLP seminar I attended in 2017. I started asking myself: *Are heart attacks really optional? Can we, as oral-health professionals, really help our patients live longer and healthier?*

The seminar was in Las Vegas, and afterward, I boarded a one-hour flight to get back home to San Jose. The last passengers to board the plane were an Asian family with two kids and a father who looked to be just a couple of years older than I was. They sat across the aisle from me. About halfway through the flight, the father stood up, walked toward the back of the plane, and collapsed. The pilot announced that the man needed medical attention, and due to the medical emergency, the plane would land as quickly as possible. Multiple people gave him CPR at the back of the plane while his wife and kids watched from afar. Although the man was given CPR for over thirty minutes, he died of a heart attack before the plane landed.

Again, he was not much older than me, and I will never forget walking off that plane and seeing his wife and children crying near the black curtains that concealed his body while they wheeled him through the airport.

That really made me think: Could a dentist who was in tune with oral-systemic disease have been integral in getting this man the proper help and education earlier in his life—possibly even preventing his death?

FROM TREAT IT AND BEAT IT TO TRANSFORMATIVE HEALTH

In the years I've spent studying the connection between a healthy mouth and a long, healthy life, I've learned that oral health is not tangential—though some people have spent their entire lives ingesting that lie. What's happening in your mouth is an excellent indicator of what's happening in the rest of the body, providing a holistic snapshot of your overall health.

The problem is, many of today's practitioners aren't interested in holistic snapshots. They're fixers, highly skilled at what I call "treat it and beat it." They want to treat the current symptoms so they can beat the disease. And while I'm all for beating disease, that approach leaves something to be desired.

To understand where this attitude came from—and why it persists—we need to first understand the growing pains that healthcare has gone through since the dawn of time. I want to introduce you to Dr. Chip Whitney, a pioneer in the field of transformative health, whose wisdom has had a powerful effect on my own complete health practice. It was Dr. Whitney who introduced me to the three eras of health identified by Dr. Lester Breslow in the *American Journal of Public Health*.[1]

The first era started at the beginning of humankind. From the shamans and medicine men, early practitioners were literally and figuratively wandering in the dark. Health providers didn't have a lot of tools, and the tools they did have often yielded the opposite result from the ones they intended. Take, for example, the doctors who leeched sick people, believing their "bad blood" was at fault—inadvertently killing their patients, who died from loss of blood.

In the early days of human history, the focus was on battling infectious diseases. These diseases killed people in staggering numbers. The bubonic plague that swept through Europe in the fourteenth century—nicknamed the "Black Death"—killed an estimated fifty million men, women, and children, which was somewhere between 25 and 60 percent of the European population.

In light of statistics like that, no wonder the first era of healthcare was about survival. Infectious diseases were claiming millions of lives, so the only thing that mattered was trying to stop them through whatever means possible.

Now fast-forward a few hundred years. By the early 1900s, medicine had made significant advances. As public health trends improved, doctors and researchers had access to new tools and treatments. They developed antibiotics, which transformed the healthcare landscape forever.

In 1956, Elvis Presley posed publicly for his polio vaccination. This came at a time when tens of thousands of children were dying from polio, and those who weren't killed were often permanently

---

1   Lester Breslow, "Health Measurement in the Third Era of Health," *Am J Public Health* 96, no. 1 (January 2006): 17–19, https://www.ncbi.nlm.nih.gov/pmc/articles/PMC1470427/.

paralyzed. Elvis's plug was highly effective; even though the vaccine had not yet been thoroughly tested, parents lined up to have their children inoculated.

Suddenly, a world that had been shrouded in darkness was exposed to the light—and the second era of healthcare began.

If the first era was about battling infectious diseases, the second era was about combating *chronic* diseases. In the latter half of the twentieth century, medicine advanced at an astonishing rate. Doctors began to identify and treat cancers. Surgery went from being a risky endeavor with terrifying instruments and a high mortality rate to a procedure that saved countless lives. Heart surgeons and brain surgeons undertook formidable challenges—and surpassed them with flying colors. Over the last fifty years, the amount of technology, medicine, and treatment options has been revolutionary.

But how does that explain people like the man on the airplane? How did a seemingly healthy man in his early forties suffer a heart attack that ended his life?

The answer is simple. The second era of healthcare, as wonderful as it is, is still fundamentally flawed. The mindset of every physician in this country is "find the disease and fix it." In other words, "treat it and beat it." It is reactionary, not proactive. It treats the patient as an amalgam of symptoms and complaints, not a unique, complex human being who needs *healthcare*, not just *sick care*.

The third era of healthcare is about *mindset*. We need a new mindset among all health professions to help our patients create health, not just react to disease. The creation of health is not just about feeling okay today. It's about feeling great tomorrow—and all the tomorrows after that.

Our goal is to take a person who is not yet sick—who may not even have developed a problem—and prevent them from ever going down a path that will create an illness.

Our main focus is simple yet powerful: *we create health.*

And who's at the cutting edge of this new third era?

We are. Your friendly neighborhood dental specialists.

> We need a new mindset among all health professions to help our patients create health, not just react to disease.

IT'S ALL CONNECTED

I'm going to tell you something you might not want to hear.

That man on the airplane could be anyone.

He could even be you.

In the human body, nothing happens in a vacuum. Everything is interconnected. But it is only now, in this third era of healthcare, that we are beginning to understand how and why.

You might be doing everything right: exercising, eating well, going in for your yearly checkups. If that's the case, more power to you. But your oral health treatment must also be looking at the bigger picture.

For years, dentistry has been associated with pain, both financial and physical. If that's the way you feel about going to see the dentist, I understand completely. Why would you willingly engage in something that only causes you pain? Only an idiot would sign up for that! I know exactly where you're coming from.

But I have good news for you. When you start thinking about dentistry in the context of complete health, it transforms from a place of pain and dread to a place of empowerment, where you, the patient, get to play an active role in your own care. Every day I partner with my patients in ways that are exciting, transformative, and even fun.

Once you embrace the mouth as the gateway to complete health, great things can happen.

When I see a patient in my practice, my goal is not to drill, fill, and bill. I'm far more interested in the bigger picture of my patient's overall health.

That's why I use a process I like to call *projection diagnostics*. *Projection diagnostics* is a fancy term for a straightforward concept. I'm trying to project the patient's future health path by using diagnostic testing technologies, such as saliva tests.

If a patient is on a bad health path, they can typically see right in front of them where their problems lie, and we can course correct. The trickier patients are the ones like the man on the airplane, people who *seem* to be healthy … but underneath the surface there's something more serious going on.

When patients first come to see me, I am determined to figure out *why* they have periodontal disease. Now, I take off my white coat and don my detective hat, ready to solve the mystery.

Even when a patient is fit, young, and healthy, I know they may be at risk for heart disease, especially if they have inflamed gums, because heart attacks are caused by inflammation, and the inflammation that leads to a heart attack has to come from somewhere.

In some cases, it's coming from a sore tooth. When I find that in a patient, I may need to send them to an endodontist for a root canal. If the endodontist discovers a badly infected tooth, then we know that the bacteria from the infection can enter the bloodstream and elicit an inflammatory reaction wherever they land, including vulnerable coronary arteries, creating the ideal conditions for a heart attack.

That's right: a tooth infection can drive vascular risk. What you might think of as a minor nuisance—a sore tooth, something a couple of ibuprofens could fix—can end your life.

THE MOUTH IS THE GATEWAY

America is the wealthiest nation in the world, yet we are one of the unhealthiest. If that surprises you, I understand. Until I shifted my focus to complete health, I didn't know all the depressing statistics—and I certainly didn't know how to change them. But there is evidence-based science to support the oral-systemic connection.

The mouth is the gateway to the body. It has key physiological functions that make it essential to our health and well-being—we eat with our mouths, we breathe through our mouths, we have immunity through our mouths. We kiss with our mouths too, and our oral health can even determine things like social status and hireability. If your teeth are badly decayed or missing entirely, you probably aren't going to get that front-row job.

For years doctors have overlooked the connection between what happens in a person's mouth and what happens in the rest of their body. The third era of healthcare requires a seismic shift. The better we understand—and care for—our oral cavity, the better chance we have of living a long, healthy life.

In this book, we're going to examine the mouth as a gateway to overall health. When bacteria from the oral cavity enter our bloodstream and spread everywhere, our body responds with inflammation, which sparks an inflammatory cascade. This cascade can lead to cardiovascular disease, dementia, cancers, sleep apnea, obesity, diabetes, and pregnancy complications—all of which we'll talk about in depth.

For each of these diseases, we'll look at the role your oral health plays and how to identify—and treat—early warning signs. Every chapter includes sections titled "The Mouth-Body Connection" and "What Can You Do about It?" This is where I'll share specific treatment options and ways to predict and prevent serious disease so that you never find yourself in a situation like the man on the plane, facing a sudden heart attack with no idea why.

I don't want you to feel scared and daunted after reading this book. I want you to feel empowered. My goal is to arm you with both the tools and strategies you need to make informed decisions about your mouth, your health, and your life.

In the pages that follow, I'll introduce you to experts and practitioners who have studied chronic disease extensively and understand the crucial role of oral health. These doctors, nurses, and researchers are paving the way for a new kind of healthcare. They have not only revolutionized the way I run *my* practice; they are leading the charge for Complete Health Dentistry® around the world.

You are standing at the precipice of the third era. Together, we have the power to transform healthcare in our world, our country, and our individual lives. True "healthcare reform" isn't political. It's about treating the whole person and taking a long view, rather than sticking a Band-Aid on as a temporary solution.

It isn't about treating and beating.

It isn't about drilling and filling.

It isn't even about dentistry.

It's about *you* and your health. I want to ensure that you are happy and healthy for many years to come.

To do that, we have to talk about the original offender: the root cause of all the diseases we'll be discussing in this book.

I'm talking about the silent assassin that could end your life at any age.

Inflammation.

CHAPTER 3

INFLAMMATION: THE SILENT KILLER

I want you to imagine a beautiful antique car in an auto show. The paint is candy-apple red, polished to a fine sheen. The interior is flawless. The owner took very good care of his prized possession, so there's not a spot of rust on it—not even when you pop the hood. The car has impeccable maintenance records, and all these years later, if you turn the keys in the ignition, the engine still purrs.

Unfortunately, we human beings are rarely so well maintained.

Maybe you've had to face one or more diseases in your life. Maybe you haven't. But either way, you are rusting. That's just part of life on this earth. The scientific term for rusting is *oxidation*, which leads to inflammation, which leads to a host of nasty diseases that range from unpleasant to fatal.

We all live in a state of chronic inflammation. That's the basis for every single disease—cardiovascular disease, dementia, cancers, and other chronic ailments. In the last chapter, I talked about the inflammatory cascade. But since the word *inflammation* can feel esoteric and hard to quantify, I like to explain it in more concrete terms.

Let's say you're chopping vegetables in the kitchen. Your hand slips, and you nick your finger with the knife. Nothing major—no need for a trip to the emergency room—but it stings, so you hold it under the faucet for a few minutes until it stops bleeding. Then you make an impromptu tourniquet out of a paper towel and go back to chopping vegetables for dinner.

For you, the cut is over.

For your body, it's only just begun.

Your skin serves as a barrier between the inside of your body and the harmful bacteria lurking on the outside: pathogens like bacteria, viruses, and other microorganisms. But now there's a break in the skin, providing a way for pathogens to enter your body. Once bacteria sneak in through the cut, they can infect the wound.

Now, your body doesn't throw in the towel at the first glimpse of bacteria. On the contrary: when tissue is injured or infected, the body mounts a solid defense, releasing chemicals that trigger an inflammatory response to kill the invaders.

You might be thinking, "Great, my body's a fighter!" And that's true—at least initially. Your body ignites its inflammatory response to solve the problem and resolve the cut, and for a day or two, your fingertip gets red and puffy and feels sore. A week later, once the body has fought the bacteria and won, your finger is as good as new.

But when the triggers of inflammation never stop, our natural functioning can go haywire. Sometimes when our bodies fight back, they don't know when to stop. This is *chronic inflammation*, which drives chronic disease.

THE WAR YOU DIDN'T KNOW YOU WERE FIGHTING

Let's talk about bacteria for a moment. These are microscopic organisms, and there are a *lot* of them. The global human population is currently around 7.6 billion, and in the volume of a single nickel you'll find 8 billion bacteria. That's right—one nickel yields more microscopic organisms than there are people on planet Earth.

There are 13 trillion bacteria in your intestines alone—so many that I've heard doctors describe them as an organ system in and of themselves. There are good bacteria and bad bacteria. When the delicate balance of the microbiome of your intestine gets out of whack and the bad outcompetes the good, it can lead to disease.

And then there's your mouth.

As we've established, the mouth is the gateway to the body. Unfortunately for your body, your mouth hosts billions of bacteria. Your tongue, teeth, and gums are bathing in bacteria at this very moment. Think about *that* next time you kiss your spouse.

Unfortunately for you, these pathogens get along fantastically with one another, so they stick together and multiply. Eventually they form a colony, and after long enough, that colony creates a thick layer of plaque. Think of plaque like very bad houseguests—they make your life a living nightmare … then stay forever.

If you've ever been to a dentist (and I hope you have), you've heard of plaque. But it's kind of like hearing the safety instructions on an airplane; after a while, we've heard the words so many times, they no longer have any meaning.

Here's what you need to know about plaque: it spreads.

And I don't mean spreads in the way syrup oozes slowly over your pancakes. Plaque spreads like wildfire, taking over your mouth, teeth, tongue, cheeks—anywhere it can reach. If it can find an opening in your mouth that takes it directly to your bloodstream, all the better. The ravenous bacteria will happily stalk the rest of our body, wreaking havoc wherever and however they can.

But your body is wise to plaque's game. It prepares a counter-attack, waging war by firing inflammatory bullets on these foreign organisms—which in turn makes the plaque fight harder. Like any high school football team, the bacteria know the best defense is a good offense, so they launch barriers of resistance against the inflammatory attack.

In other words, there's a microscopic war raging inside you—and you have no idea.

You have a chronic inflammatory bacterial condition in your mouth. Chronic means your body never turns off the process of inflammation. It's like cutting your finger over and over and over again. The body is beleaguered by the constant assault of bacteria without an opportunity to resolve it, so the inflammatory response never powers down. What happens then?

You get sick.

THE DEADLY DANCE

As a part of his research on complete health transformation, Dr. Chip Whitney talks about three kinds of "body pollution" that lead to disease. Just like there is pollution in the air, pollution in the body drives people down certain chronic disease paths. For Dr. Whitney, the three main pollutants are oxidative stress, free radicals, and—you guessed it—inflammation.

At this point you may be thinking, "I'm strong and healthy. I've never had a serious health problem or disease. Who's to say my body won't be able to fight off bacteria without causing chronic inflammation?"

In a perfect world, your body would do just that. But this isn't a perfect world. If the cause of inflammation never stops, inflammation never turns off. The reality is that our bodies get worn down over time. We rust.

> If the cause of inflammation never stops, inflammation never turns off. The reality is that our bodies get worn down over time.

Some of the root causes of body pollution are minimally under our control. Take, for example, genetics and family history. We all have genetic predispositions to certain diseases, whether we like it or not. Then there's gut dysbiosis, where once again bad bacteria begin to dominate the good bacteria and throw everything out of balance. Insulin resistance, sleep apnea, high visceral (belly) fat—these are some of the root causes of pollution, and pollution is the root cause of disease.

It's important to note here that not all diseases are alike. In the last chapter, we talked about the bubonic plague, which we now know was caused by a single bacterium. Many illnesses can be traced back to one bacterium, including those that *didn't* cause sweeping epidemics, such as strep throat or pneumonia.

What I'm talking about is not a single bacterium. I'm talking about the massive hordes of bacteria that build up in the mouth and lower intestines and are dangerous because of *quantity*, not quality. Just one of them isn't going to cause a problem, but together they drive the infection. En masse, they creep into the bloodstream, triggering inflammation that can be transmitted to other organs.

Chronic inflammation is the root cause of almost all chronic disease. But there's one root cause of inflammation we haven't touched on. I saved the best for last.

Periodontal disease.

A.k.a., gum disease.

As a periodontist, I see a lot of gum disease. I have a front-row seat to inflammation in the tissues of the mouth. It starts as gingivitis, when your gums become swollen and red and may even bleed. As the disease progresses into full-blown periodontitis, the gums can pull away from the tooth, leading to bone loss and lost teeth.

Do you see how everything is connected? It all begins with bacteria, which causes periodontal disease. The pathogens trigger the body's inflammatory response, which in turn leads to inflammation in the mouth as the body tries to fight back. The mouth is the body's gateway, so the bacteria get into the bloodstream and spread everywhere, landing in the organs, the brain, and the arteries along the way, driving the same inflammation in those distant sites that is already present in the oral cavity.

And that, my friends, is a delicate, deadly dance that drives chronic disease.

THE THREE WAR ZONES

In the following chapters, we'll take a closer look at the three most worrisome diseases that result from inflammation. We'll start with cardiovascular disease, which covers heart attacks and strokes. A stroke is exactly the same as a heart attack, only it's a brain attack instead: same process, different location.

Then we'll talk about dementia and Alzheimer's disease. After that, we'll discuss various cancers, including colorectal, pancreatic, and esophageal. We'll also look at the interplay between inflammation and sleep apnea, obesity, diabetes, and pregnancy complications.

> There are ways to transform your health *before you ever get sick.*

Here's my promise to you: this book is not all gloom and doom. There are ways to transform your health *before you ever get sick.* That's why every chapter ends with one simple question: "What Can You Do about It?" For each disease, I will share treatment options and other helpful resources. I want to show you how to change the path you're on before you end up at a destination you never want to visit.

The first step is to educate ourselves. If we don't know what we're looking for, we won't know how to fight it.

I'm a periodontist, so I see all kinds of things in my practice. One thing that continues to amaze me is how many of my new patients tell me their gums bleed when they brush their teeth.

"Just a little," they say. "Nothing major."

I want you to think about this for a moment. The total area of your gums is about the size of the palm of your hand. If you looked at the palm of your hand and saw an open wound, would you do something about it? Or would you continue to let it bleed?

Bleeding gums means there's an infection. Something is definitely wrong. But many people don't see it that way. They just spit a little blood and toothpaste into their bathroom sink in the morning and go on with their day.

The problem is, the mouth is only the beginning. Periodontal disease doesn't stop in your gums. Inflammation in the gums allows bacteria to spew into other parts of the body. Your organs. Your brain. Your heart.

Remember the man on the airplane who died from a heart attack? Based on his age, gender, genetic history, and general health and fitness, he may have appeared to be low risk but was, instead, harboring silent vascular disease. That can be caused by inflammation from the mouth that travels through arteries, causing a blockage of blood flow to the heart.

Which leads me to the question we've all been dying to ask: Is there anything we can do to prevent it?

STRAIGHT TO THE HEART

At the beginning of this chapter, I asked you to imagine a mint-condition antique car at an auto show. Now I want you to envision yourself at ninety years old. What do you see? Do you see a polished antique automobile with an engine that still purrs? Or do you see a rusty old mess when you pop the hood?

If you want to be healthy and happy at ninety, you need a healthy body and a healthy brain. You should be able to be as independent and active as you want to be. To get there, you need a strategy.

Most people don't have a strategy. We have plenty of strategies about our careers, finances, professional achievements, friendships, and even romantic relationships. But when we think about creating health, we tend to think in terms of losing weight, exercising, and eating well. That's it.

Those are *tools* to creating health, not strategies. At the heart of any good health strategy is identifying early disease. That's essential, because it is chronic disease that can steal life span from even the healthiest of individuals.

Identifying early disease can be challenging, especially when that disease is asymptomatic—as it usually is. Most of us do this in some form or another already; we schedule mammograms to screen for breast cancer, colonoscopies to screen for colon cancer, and so on. Lucky for us, twenty-first-century technology is rapidly evolving, increasing our ability to identify disease at an early treatable state.

The problem is that many diseases are untreatable once discovered.

So what do we do?

The answer is simple: we have to prevent the untreatable disease. We have to make the impossible possible. And the way to do that is by connecting the dots. We can prevent disease by reverse engineering our way back to the inflammation that causes it in the first place.

The best way to start, of course, is to go straight to the heart.

CHAPTER 4

THE HEART OF THE MATTER

If I asked you to tell me the number-one killer in this country, what would you say?

Car accidents?

Cancer?

The answer—which you've probably guessed from the chapter title—is heart disease.

Cardiovascular disease is the leading cause of death and disability for both men and women in the United States. Here's another statistic that will blow your mind: recent research has found that oral infections can trigger up to *50 percent or more of acute heart attacks*!

> Prevention can start in the dentist's chair.

That number is staggering, and it means people like the man on the airplane are far from unique. The current cost of cardiovascular disease to our healthcare system is about $518 billion. And guess what?

I believe it's preventable.

Prevention can start in the dentist's chair. But before we look at the link between a healthy mouth and a healthy heart, we have to understand how cardiovascular disease works—and why it's so dangerous.

OUT, DAMNED CLOT!

Cardiovascular disease is the umbrella term for a number of different events in the body, including the following:

- Aneurysm

- Angina

- Atherosclerosis

- Cerebrovascular accident (stroke)

- Cerebrovascular disease

- Congestive heart failure

- Coronary artery disease

- Electrical malfunctions like atrial fibrillation

- Myocardial infarction (heart attack)

- Peripheral vascular disease

- Valve diseases

In the last chapter we talked about plaque in the mouth, the nightmare houseguest nobody would ever want. In the arteries (the blood vessels supplying oxygen to the heart), plaque can cause a narrowing that makes it harder for blood to flow. If someone is harboring silent plaque in their body, and the plaque ruptures like a volcano in the inner lining of the artery, it's bad news all around. That is a heart attack. If it occurs in the carotid artery in our neck, it causes a stroke or transient ischemic attack.

Remember how our bodies are trying so hard to protect us? When plaque ruptures the wall of an artery, our body says, "We better heal that injury!" In the same way a scab forms over the wound when a kid skins their knee, your body automatically sends a clotting cascade to heal the rupture of the artery wall.

If you shiver at the word *clotting*, you should. A heart attack occurs when the blood flow to a part of the heart is blocked by a blood clot. If the clot cuts off the blood flow completely, the part of the heart muscle supplied by that artery begins to die.

This event usually occurs in a small blockage. Eighty-six percent of heart attacks occur from the rupture of a plaque so small that it would not have resulted in an abnormal stress test. Some of you may remember NBC News anchor Tim Russert. Tim had a completely normal stress test in April 2008. He died of a heart attack in June 2008. It was not that he had a bad doctor or a bad test; he just had a small plaque that did not show up on testing. A stress test is simply not an effective screening test.

In an ischemic stroke—which accounts for about 85 percent of strokes—the process is exactly the same; it just happens in a different location. The word *ischemic* comes from the Greek *iskhaimos*, or "stopping blood." If the blood clot blocks blood flow in the heart, we call it a heart attack. If it floats from the carotid artery in our neck and lands in the brain, we call it a stroke. When the blood supply to a part of the brain is shut off, brain cells will die, impeding normal functions such as walking or talking.

Some of us are genetically predisposed to heart disease, and we can't change the genes we inherited. But there is one place where we can exercise a great deal of control.

You guessed it.

Our mouths.

THE MOUTH-ARTERY CONNECTION

As usual, the culprit is inflammation.

When oral bacteria enter the bloodstream and reach arteries, these arteries can incur the body's inflammatory wrath. The same inflammatory response that causes bleeding gums will occur in the walls of a vulnerable artery. Inflammation may cause the artery to rupture, then form a clot as the natural effort to heal the rupture, and as you know, that can result in a heart attack or stroke.

There's a good deal of hard science on the link between oral health and heart disease. Studies published in prominent medical journals like *Circulation*, *Journal of the American Heart Association*, and *Lancet* have shown the connection between infection in the mouth and cerebrovascular and cardiovascular disease. Major universities and medical institutions like the Cleveland Clinic are already changing their standard of care to incorporate the oral-systemic associations that research has uncovered.

Take, for example, the study done on 1,163 men showing the oral bacterium *Porphyromonas gingivalis* to be associated with coronary heart disease.[2] The same scientists went back and performed an even larger study of 6,950 subjects, providing serological evidence that an infection caused by major periodontal pathogens increased the risk

---

2   P. J. Pussinen, P. Jousilahti, G. Alfthan, T. Palosuo, S. Asikainen, and V. Salomaa, "Antibodies to Periodontal Pathogens Are Associated with Coronary Heart Disease," *Arterioscler Thromb Vasc Biol* 23 (2003): 1,250–1,254.

of future stroke.[3] Several years later, the National Institutes of Health supported a third study in which researchers detected invasive periodontal pathogens at the sites of atherosclerotic disease.[4] Bacterial presence in the artery wall was actually demonstrated through DNA technology.

In other words, a significant contributor to the plaque that built up in the walls of the patient's arteries had originated in his mouth!

Further investigative work needs to be performed, as is always the case with evidence-based research. But these studies—and numerous others—have established an unequivocal link. Now that we understand this important contributor to cardiovascular disease, we're able to develop novel therapies for treating it.

Of course, there will always be naysayers. In a recent guest editorial to the *Journal of the American Dental Association* (JADA), Dr. Bruce L. Pihlstrom called into question the oral-systemic link, saying, "There remains a need for more convincing and higher quality evidence that oral healthcare actually has a measurable impact on specific systemic diseases before it can be claimed that attaining good oral health can prevent systemic diseases or conditions."[5]

The response from the American Academy for Oral Systemic Health (AAOSH) was swift and mighty. The AAOSH board wrote a

---

3   P. J. Pussinen, G. Alfthan, H. Rissanen, A. Reunanen, S. Asikainen, and P. Knekt, "Antibodies to Periodontal Pathogens and Stroke Risk," *Stroke* 35 (2004): 2,020–2,023.

4   E. V. Kozarov, B. R. Dorn, C. E. Shelburne, W. A. Dunn, and A. Progulske-Fox, "Human Atherosclerotic Plaque Contains Viable Invasive *Actinobacillus actinomycetemcomitans* and *Porphyromonas gingivalis*," *Arteriosclerosis, Thrombosis, and Vascular Biology* 25 (2005): e17–e18.

5   B. Pihlstrom, J. Hodges, B. Michalowicz, J. C. Wohlfahrt, and R. Garcia, "Promoting Oral Health Care Because of Its Possible Effect on Systemic Disease Is Premature and May Be Misleading," *JADA* 149 (2018): 401–403.

position paper in which it called out JADA for its myopic, old-school thinking and failure to see the bigger picture.

"A little over a decade ago," the paper states, "we had no idea that the complexity of periodontal disease was enough to negatively influence glycemic control or cardiovascular health. But it is a disservice to unknowing patients when practitioners neglect the mounting associations, causation, and level-A evidence that infection in the mouth significantly contributes to medical conditions like heart attacks, stroke, Alzheimer's disease, cancers, diabetes, pre-term births, and a host of other inflammatory conditions."[6]

As my friends and colleagues at the AAOSH noted, "Change is never easy. But the evidence of a significant association between oral and systemic health is incontrovertible. We must not let the complexity of this association deter us from expanding the nature and scope of our care when it is so clearly warranted."

As Dr. Whitney pointed out in his 2012 editorial published in *Dentistry Today*, "There is absolutely no risk to optimal dental care and home oral hygiene … What is the repercussion if we assume oral bacteria do not contribute to vascular disease and we are wrong? We miss the opportunity to significantly impact the lives of millions of people on the path to suffer a cardiovascular event!"

WOMEN WITH HEALTHY HEARTS

I want to introduce you to Dr. Gina Pritchard, cardiovascular nurse practitioner and the founder and director of the Prevent Clinic. For Dr. Pritchard, heart attacks and strokes are *not* an inevitable part of

---

6   J. Russo, S. Estep, S. Maples, D. Wilkerson, M. Milligan, V. Richards, J. Lazarus et al., "AAOSH Responds to *JADA* Editorial That Claims Promoting Oral-Systemic Connection Is 'Premature and Misleading,'" *American Academy for Oral Systemic Health*, June 15, 2018, https://aaosh.org/jada-response.

life. She travels and speaks as an advocate for early detection and prevention of heart disease, educating people everywhere on the importance of heart health.

We often think of breast cancer as the biggest health concern for women. Most of us know a woman who has fought it, and we see the signature pink ribbons everywhere we look. The whole month of October is dedicated to breast cancer awareness. And for good reason: one in thirty women will die of breast cancer.

It may surprise you to hear that *one in three* women will die of cardiovascular disease.

The PR campaign for detecting cardiovascular disease could learn a thing or two from breast cancer, because if heart disease had the same name recognition, thousands of lives might be saved. And yet cardiovascular disease kills more men and women than all kinds of cancer combined.

Dr. Pritchard has found that many people think of cardiovascular disease as a "man's disease," which simply isn't true. Heart attacks happen to just as many women as men, though they happen on average ten years later.

Women also have a different set of risk factors to contend with. For example, polycystic ovary syndrome (PCOS) is a hormonal disorder common among women. PCOS is a genetically driven type of insulin resistance that also increases the risk of cardiovascular disease. If you are a woman with PCOS—or if you have a wife, sister, mother, or daughter with PCOS—early screening is all the more essential.

Because women often experience different symptoms of cardiovascular disease than men, it can sometimes be harder to detect. In the months before a heart attack, a woman might be unusually fatigued—which they could just as easily chalk up to a bad night of sleep. They might also experience indigestion, weak arms, a racing heart, or anxiety. While a man might complain of gripping chest pains during a heart attack, women can have subtler, less recognizable symptoms, such as nausea; pain or discomfort in the back, stomach, jaw, or neck; and shortness of breath. Because women are often unaware these symptoms might mean a heart attack or cardiovascular disease, they ignore the signs.

"I give a female twist to the complete health workup," Dr. Pritchard says. "Not just in the dental office, but the collaborative practice model where the dental community, dental team, and the medical team are working together in an integrated approach. We want to screen, appropriately diagnose, and then either treat existing cardiovascular disease or prevent early stage atherosclerosis from developing. We can prevent an event in the future for patients with or without existing cardiovascular disease."

Dr. Pritchard believes strongly in early-stage screening. She goes around the country championing the carotid intima-media thickness ultrasound, which is being performed in more and more dental offices—and rightly so. "I did my doctoral work on early screening," Pritchard says, "and it's something that I'm helping dentists, dental hygienists, MDs, DOs, and nurse practitioners with in offices all across the United States." She hopes to expand to other countries, too, as Complete Health Dentistry® goes global.

Preventing cardiovascular disease *is* possible—but you won't know how to treat it if you don't know where to look.

WHAT CAN YOU DO ABOUT IT?

Here's the good news: unlike many other chronic medical conditions, cardiovascular disease is treatable and can be reversible, even after a long history of disease.

The first step is detection. As Dr. Gina Pritchard and Dr. Chip Whitney can attest, early screening could save your life. That vital journey might begin with a trip to the dentist—as long as your dentist is an advocate and practitioner of Complete Health Dentistry®.

I want to introduce you to Brad Bale, MD, and Amy Doneen, MSN, ARNP, DNP. Ten years ago, when Dr. Bale and Dr. Doneen first started working together, they began to investigate the oral-systemic link. They learned that, although there are many pathologies that drive vascular events, oral health doesn't seem to get enough attention in the medical world. The more they looked into the data and literature, the more convinced they were that the same bacteria that cause periodontal disease also cause heart attacks and ischemic strokes.

So why wasn't oral health getting enough credit? Because the medical and dental communities just did not understand. They decided to take matters into their own hands.

Together, the doctors founded the BaleDoneen Method® for preventing heart attacks, strokes, and type II diabetes. Now they teach physicians, dentists, and other healthcare providers around the world their method for early detection and treatment.

For Dr. Bale and Dr. Doneen, a critical component of early detection and treatment is simple: go to the dentist, get your teeth and gums evaluated regularly, and accept the recommended treatment plan when you need to—not just so you can have pretty teeth, but because it might save your life.

"Periodontal disease is extremely prevalent," says Dr. Bale. "Once you're thirty years of age, there's a 50 percent chance you have it. Once you're sixty-five, there's an 80 percent chance. If you don't want to have a heart attack or stroke, you need to maintain a healthy mouth, be evaluated thoroughly for periodontal disease, and if it's present, eradicate it."[7]

Dr. Bale and Dr. Doneen are so confident in their work that they actually guarantee it: since 2008, they have offered all patients treated at their clinics—the Heart Attack and Stroke Prevention Center in Spokane, Washington, and the Heart Attack, Stroke, and Diabetes Center at the Grace Clinic in Lubbock, Texas—a written guarantee stating that if the patient suffers a heart attack or stroke while under their care, the doctors will refund 100 percent of the fees paid during the year.

"We get extremely high-risk patients," says Dr. Bale, "which is fine. I like a challenging patient, and I do believe you can shut down the disease process in anybody."

Dr. Bale and Dr. Doneen have worked tirelessly to synthesize all the data and develop the BaleDoneen Method®, because they truly believe that heart attacks and strokes are preventable. You can read more about their work at baledoneen.com.

In my practice, we have regular protocols for saving peoples' lives. In the first consultation, we start by taking the patient's blood pressure. We also take it at the time of surgery—that's something many practices simply don't do. But it's something that has had life-saving results.

---

7   Brad Bale and Amy Doneen, "The Vital Importance of the Mouth-Body Connection," *Oral Systemic Link*, accessed April 20, 2017, http://oralsystemiclink.net/patients/profile/the-vital-importance-of-the-mouth-body-connection.

I had performed implant surgery on Julie, and she was very happy with her outcome. A few months after we completed her case, she called us because her boyfriend was having some tooth pain. The two of them came into the office expecting him to undergo an extraction. Indeed, his x-rays revealed an infection in his tooth and the reason for his discomfort. He was all in to get the extraction done right then and there. But when we took his blood pressure, it was over 200/100! This young man was in his midthirties and had not had a medical exam in many years. He thought he was healthy; he never had a second thought that he had any medical issues.

We put him on an antibiotic, gave him pain meds, and told him to go straight to the ER that day! He was reluctant at first, but his girlfriend, who trusted us, urged him to go.

About two weeks later, he was back in our office and ready for the extraction after having been cleared by his medical doctor, who prescribed medication for him.

When I came into the operatory, he thanked me for saving his life. His doctor had informed the young man that he was at high risk for a stroke or heart attack if he had not gone to the hospital that day. We extracted his tooth, relieving his pain and getting the infection out of his mouth. It was a great day for everyone, and he was much healthier for making the trip to the dentist.

What would have happened if we had not taken his blood pressure in that first visit? When we gave him an injection, he could have had a stroke! It was not the first—or last—time that we saved a life with a simple blood pressure test. Every week, we refuse treatment to patients who are medically compromised, and most of the time, it's because of their high blood pressure.

In addition to staying on top of your periodontal care, here are some other ways to minimize your risk of having a stroke or heart attack:

- Control high blood pressure (hypertension).

- Identify inflammatory cholesterol and prediabetes early.

- Follow good oral-health maintenance practices that promote healthy gums and teeth.

- Quit tobacco use.

- Eliminate inflammatory visceral (belly) fat.

- Eat a diet rich in fruits and vegetables.

- Exercise regularly.

- Drink alcohol in moderation, if at all.

- Know your genetics.

- Establish and maintain gut health.

- Check with a provider who understands the oral-systemic connection and can evaluate you for sleep apnea and send you for testing, if needed.

The following are resources that might be helpful:

- http://www.heart.org
- http://www.periodontal.com
- http://www.news-medical.net
- http://www.perio.org
- http://oralsystemiclink.net
- https://aaosh.org/
- http://www.RHSLiveWell.com

WHAT'S NEXT?

Now that we've talked about heart health, it's time to move onward and upward. Because your mouth doesn't only tell us a lot about your cardiovascular health; it also tells us all about your brain.

CHAPTER 5

DON'T FORGET

If you've ever watched a mind deteriorate from Alzheimer's, you know it's a heartbreaking disease. It progresses quickly, and people with advanced Alzheimer's can experience major personality changes and loss of memory, so much so that they forget their own friends and family. I want to thank my associate, Dr. Lynna Bui, for sharing the following heartbreaking story about her father who died of Alzheimer's disease and other complications.

> *Our family first noticed symptoms of my father's absentmindedness in 1997. He was then diagnosed with Alzheimer's disease in 1998, when he was merely sixty years old. Initially, he would ask us the same questions repeatedly many times. Then gradually, he would not remember what day of the week it was; he would forget his daily tasks at work. One morning, he took a walk and could not find his way home; hours later, a policeman found him miles*

away from our house and brought him home to us from the address on his wrist. We all knew that he was slowly losing his memory, but we did not realize how rapidly the disease had progressed. My father was a great mathematician who started teaching during his early years, never needing to memorize any equations as he was able to quickly derive them. He was gifted and brilliant, able to recite a poem at any moment appropriate for that specific situation.

When he started to realize how forgetful he had become, he would write in his journal who he was and what he did every day, so that he would remember when he read his own writings. However, eventually his memory faded to a point that he did not recognize even his own handwriting. It was despondent and painful for us to see that he just stared at us blankly and had no clue who we were. My mother was the last one he failed to recognize. I could only imagine that my mother must have felt dejected because he was so pugnacious with her—the one who had been taking care of him daily, even the most rudimentary chores. But she never got mad at my father. He was very frustrated and combative because he did not know who he was. In early 2007, his health declined drastically. With complications of diabetes and chronic obstructive pulmonary disease (COPD), he finally passed away at sixty-nine years old, leaving us behind with intense anguish.

If you're one of the lucky few who has never had a friend or family member with Alzheimer's, chances are your luck won't last forever. An estimated eight million Americans live with Alzheimer's dementia (AD)—also known as senile dementia of the Alzheimer's type—and that number is expected to grow to *fourteen million* by 2050.[8]

Put another way, someone in the United States develops AD every sixty-five seconds. By midcentury, someone in the US will develop the disease every thirty-three seconds.

The face of Alzheimer's may not be what you think. Early-onset AD is becoming more prevalent, so that while the vast majority of people facing the disease are still over sixty-five, some are younger. In 2018, approximately two hundred thousand individuals under age sixty-five had early-onset Alzheimer's.[9]

Many of us fear we are headed toward a future of forgetting the people we love—especially those of us who've watched friends and family members decimated by this cruel, devastating disease. I won't lie to you—the statistics aren't encouraging. According to the Alzheimer's Association, "Alzheimer's disease is the only top 10 cause of death in the United States that cannot be prevented, cured, or even slowed."[10] This is arguably the most important disease Dr. Whitney refers to when he says we must prevent the untreatable.

The *good* news is that times are changing. There are an increasing number of studies suggesting what causes it. The more we learn about AD, the better chance we have of learning how to take precautionary measures to help protect us *before* it strikes.

Scientists and researchers have made—and continue to make—exciting new discoveries in the study of AD that point to the link between AD and inflammation. The field of research is still young, and more studies are needed to yield conclusive results. But the

---

8   "Fact and Figures," Alzheimer's Association, accessed November 23, 2019, https://www.alz.org/alzheimers-dementia/facts-figures.

9   "Fact and Figures," Alzheimer's Association.

10 "Facts and Figures," Alzheimer's Association.

research suggests that exposure to inflammation early in life can *quadruple* one's risk of developing Alzheimer's disease later on.

First, let's talk about what Alzheimer's is, what it isn't, and how this brutal disease has left scientists scratching their heads for a very long time.

IS ALZHEIMER'S THE SAME AS DEMENTIA?

You've probably heard "Alzheimer's disease" and "dementia" used interchangeably. The reason for this confusion may be your doctor's fault. The word *Alzheimer's* tends to evoke fear and panic, so some physicians will use the term *dementia* instead. They're not entirely wrong. Alzheimer's is one *type* of dementia. But they're not synonymous.

According to the National Institute of Neurological Disorders and Stroke (NINDS), dementia is a group of symptoms caused by disorders that affect the brain. It is not a specific disease.

NINDS goes on to say, "People with dementia may not be able to think well enough to do normal activities like getting dressed or eating. They may lose their ability to solve problems or control their emotions. Their personalities may change. They may become agitated or see things that are not there."[11]

If you find yourself thinking, "Those symptoms sound like Alzheimer's symptoms," you would be correct. There are several types of dementia, but Alzheimer's is the most common. AD is a neurodegenerative disorder defined by the Alzheimer's Foundation of America as "a progressive, degenerative disorder that attacks the brain's nerve cells, or neurons, resulting in loss of memory, loss of thinking and language skills, and behavioral changes."

---

11 "Dementia vs Alzheimer's," Fisher Center for Alzheimer's Research Foundation, accessed July 5, 2019, http://www.alzinfo.org/understand-alzheimers/dementia/.

Fun fact: AD was named after a German physician, Alois Alzheimer, who first described it in 1906. Sometimes I wonder how Alois would feel if he knew his name was known the whole world over but was associated with dread and fear. Maybe an incurable disease is *not* the way you want to be remembered.

> Since the brain runs so many of the body's operations, when your brain powers down, you power down too.

As more and more nerve cells die, Alzheimer's disease leads to significant brain shrinkage. And since the brain runs so many of the body's operations, when your brain powers down, you power down too.

The symptoms of Alzheimer's can vary in severity and chronology. But the overall progress of the disease is fairly predictable. AD is terminal: on average, people live eight to ten years after diagnosis, though they can sometimes live up to twenty. In the later stages, autonomic functions like heart rate, breathing, digestion, and autoimmune response are affected.

While the disease is fatal, it's often secondary illnesses that cause death, everything from heart attacks to kidney failure to pneumonia. Advanced Alzheimer's patients are usually too frail, their immune systems too compromised, to fight off bacterial infections that a healthier person could survive.

ALZHEIMER'S AND INFLAMMATION: A STICKY BOND

There's a lot of debate about what causes Alzheimer's disease, and the various theories often get contentious. Most scientists will concede that Alzheimer's results from a combination of genetic, lifestyle, and environmental factors that affect the brain over decades.

One thing we can all agree on is that there is plaque in the brains of Alzheimer's patients. As a dentist, I obviously talk a lot about plaque. But whereas plaque in your mouth is made up of sticky deposits between your teeth, neurological plaques are abnormal clusters of protein fragments that gum up and block the functioning of brain cells. It's like what would happen if you spilled soda on your laptop; the sticky liquid would gum up the circuitry and ruin your computer. The plaque spreads through the cortex in a predictable pattern as the disease progresses.

Where the plaque comes from—and why it so viciously attacks the brain's nerve cells—remains something of a mystery. Despite the billions of dollars that have been invested to crack the case, scientists are still not certain.

"We have done absolutely nothing to change the course of the disease," says Dr. Garth Ehrlich, a professor at Drexel University College of Medicine. "Other chronic diseases, we have affected, because we understand what causes them. There is nothing new you can do for an Alzheimer's patient that you couldn't do twenty years ago."[12]

Dr. Ehrlich isn't the only one who feels that the direction of Alzheimer's research needs to be rerouted. His colleague Dr. Herbert Allen, chair of Drexel's Department of Dermatology, became fascinated by research showing a link between Alzheimer's and bacteria in the brain. He pored over the work done by Swiss researcher Judith Miklossy, who found two types of spirochetes—long, corkscrew-

12   Lauren Ingeno, "Do Infections Cause Alzheimer's Disease?" *Drexel University News Blog*, accessed July 5, 2019, https://newsblog.drexel.edu/2016/02/10/do-infections-cause-alzheimers-disease/.

shaped bacteria—in the brains of more than 90 percent of Alzheimer's disease patients.[13] Her research suggested that most of these spirochetes originated from the mouth. Miklossy's paper, published in 2011, was soon corroborated by other studies that found a connection between bacteria and dementia.

In 2016, Dr. Allen conducted his own study. He and his team of scientists investigated seven postmortem brains of patients with Alzheimer's disease, comparing them to ten healthy brains. The results suggested that spirochetes in the brain could be creating biofilms, films of bacteria that are slimy, glue like, and incredibly resistant to antibiotics.

When he published the results of his study in *Neuroinfectious Diseases*, Dr. Allen hypothesized that "spirochetes enter the brain during a dental procedure or after a person contracts Lyme, and then spin out a protective biofilm. The body's first responders try to clear the infection, but … the immune system ends up destroying the surrounding tissue."[14]

According to Dr. Allen, the cause of Alzheimer's disease may be the body's own immune system mounting an inflammatory defense—one that could be triggered by a dental procedure or chronic inflammation of the gums.

Sound familiar?

Make no mistake, Dr. Allen's hypothesis is highly controversial. The traditional medical community loves to discredit researchers who find proof of a connection between dementia and oral health.

---

13   Judith. J. Miklossy, "Alzheimer's Disease – A Neurospirochetosis" *J. Neuroinflammation* 8, no. 90 (August 2011), https://www.ncbi.nlm.nih.gov/pubmed/21816039.

14   H. Allen, "Alzheimer's Disease: A Novel Hypothesis Integrating Spirochetes, Biofilm, and the Immune System," *J. Neuroinfectious Diseases* 7, no. 1 (2016), https://www.ncbi.nlm.nih.gov/pmc/articles/PMC5008232/.

Further research is certainly needed to confirm that spirochetal bacteria—or any bacteria—can trigger the inflammatory cascade that leads to Alzheimer's disease.

But as more research is done on the link between bacteria and Alzheimer's, I believe we'll see increasing evidence of the crucial importance of a healthy mouth. Spirochetes, the offending bacteria, are found in the oral cavity. That's a fact. And since spirochetal infection occurs years or even decades before dementia manifests, a patient could potentially prevent and eradicate Alzheimer's years before it began. Remember Dr. Whitney's comment, "What if we assume oral bacteria do not contribute to disease and are wrong?" This applies to Alzheimer's disease too. We have an opportunity to prevent the untreatable.

WHAT CAN YOU DO ABOUT IT?

Since there are currently no medically sanctioned ways to prevent Alzheimer's disease, this is a tricky question. Since the research on neuroinflammation is new and growing, we're still wandering in the dark.

But there is light at the end of the tunnel, as scientists and researchers begin to illuminate the path. Dr. Dale Bredesen, a professor of neurology at the David Geffen School of Medicine at UCLA, recently launched a yearslong study on ten patients with AD.[15] The results of the study, published in the journal *Aging*, were landmark, the first to suggest that memory loss in patients *may in fact be reversed*. Bredesen used a complex, thirty-six-point therapeutic program that involved comprehensive diet changes, brain stimu-

---

15   Mark Wheeler, "Memory Loss Associated with Alzheimer's Reversed for First Time," *UCLA Newsroom*, accessed July 5, 2019, http://newsroom.ucla.edu/releases/memory-loss-associated-with-alzheimers-reversed-for-first-time.

lation, exercise, sleep optimization, specific pharmaceuticals and vitamins, and multiple additional steps that affect brain chemistry.

For me, the results of Bredesen's work are encouraging. I believe an inflammatory burden early in life, as represented by chronic periodontal disease, could have severe consequences later as a contributing factor to Alzheimer's. If the link between inflammation and Alzheimer's disease is confirmed, researchers say it would add reducing inflammatory burden to the short list of preventable risk factors for Alzheimer's disease.

As you may recall, in the first chapter, I mentioned how airway and sleep can affect Alzheimer's. That is vital information that I learned from Dr. Whitney, who also taught me about fasting. Today I also know, thanks to a deep understanding of the oral-systemic connection, that diabetics are at higher risk of getting AD. They are also at higher risk of getting periodontal disease, and inflammation from periodontal disease is also connected to Alzheimer's. It's all connected.

What does all of this mean for you?

It means go to your dentist regularly, accept the recommended treatment plan to reduce the bacterial load in your mouth, and do everything in your power to combat inflammation when—or better yet, *before*—it strikes.

The following are some resources that might be helpful:

- http://www.medicalnewstoday.com
- https://www.brightfocus.org/alzheimers
- https://www.alz.org/alzheimers-dementia/what-is-alzheimers/
- https://www.drbredesen.com/thebredesenprotocol

WHAT'S NEXT?

We've talked about cardiovascular health and brain health—how inflammation can lead to a heart attack and might even cause brain cells to die.

But what about other systems of the body? Does inflammation cause widespread health problems in organs like your colon or your lungs?

You bet it does. In the next chapter, I'll explain how.

CHAPTER 6

AN INFLAMED BODY
IS A SICK BODY

My cousin Bradley recently shared with me what it was like to watch his mother lose her battle with cancer.

Mom absolutely loved the Christmas season. After all, she was born in December, the eleventh day to be exact. She lit up at just the thought of the time of year when the city is decked out with lights, ribbons, and that giving spirit. She'd spend hours, days, weeks decorating the house and crafting with her glue gun, meticulously securing each ornament to her wreaths and tabletop tree displays. The year 2017 was a little different. Creating and the sound of Christmas music in the house started in early August, a couple of months after we received the horrible news of inoperable pancreatic cancer, and not even a year after we lost dad to cancer. Also, the thought of her mom, my grandma, lasting six months, and her older sister just three months after hearing the same diagnosis, weighed heavily on all of us. We knew immersing herself in the season was how she was coping with it all. She went where she could escape, to what she loved and enjoyed losing herself in.

On December 15, four days after Mom's eighty-third birthday, five of her very best friends gathered upstairs at home around her. Lining the edge of her hospital bed we had brought in, we sang "Happy Birthday" as she beamed a very appreciative smile. This was after eighteen months and countless trips to the doctor. My lively, active, thoughtful, and loving mom lay bedridden, a skeletal frame of a once healthy, happy, beautiful person.

"Please, please, Bradley, I just want it to end, please help meee, pleeease." Mom pleaded in a weak though very decisive tone, as she glanced at me and grimaced in pain.

"I wish I could, Mom. I can't do anything. I really wish I could do something," I replied.

I sat beside her, holding her hand, mom's nurse at the foot of her bed and one of her longtime friends next to me. Thirty minutes or so passed, the oxygen tanks just delivered, and it was time to change her bedding and give her a sponge bath.

"I want to get out of this bed," Mom said suddenly and firmly. We all looked at each other surprised, though I understood her request. "Can you just roll me down the hall?" she asked.

We knew it would be a challenge getting her from the bed into the chair, since she was still quite heavy and unable to assist at all. But she was adamant that she wanted to get up, and I agreed, of course. It was early evening, not quite dark yet, when the three of us started to position her, first raising her upper body with the hospital bed, then her legs off the side of the bed toward me. We got her to sit up, and I placed myself in front of her, my arms under hers.

"Okay, you ready, Mom?" I said.

"Yes," she said.

Then I squatted a bit and lifted her up as the nurse held the wheelchair to keep it in place. I heard a clicking sound from inside Mom, and she gasped. I knew something had just happened as I lowered her into the chair. Her breathing became rapid and larger, her eyes glassy and fixed until she took one last big breath. I called for my wife, who was tending to our little one downstairs. We put our arms around Mom and said our goodbyes before making the calls to family and friends. At the end, I had helped my mom as she pleaded with me to do earlier that day. It was ironically the last act I did for her during her life.

Of course, I was very sad and upset but relieved that she was no longer suffering. I had no regrets as I had done all I could with my own hands and heart. We had taken one last trip to Japan two months prior to visit my in-laws. I wheeled Mom through literally every aisle of at least a dozen Daiso-100 Yen stores in Osaka. I had danced with her at my—her only child's—wedding three months after her diagnosis. We celebrated her one and only grandson's first birthday. A lot had happened within the previous eighteen months, and before that, she had felt like she was just getting started, hopeful that she'd be enjoying grandchildren and *passing on her famous baking recipes and techniques to her new daughter-in-law.*

In the normal process of grieving after receiving the news, she had expressed her anger at the start of her diagnosis. She was angry that her doctor seemingly dismissed her concern when she asked to run tests to check on the condition of her pancreas, despite her family history. She was angry at herself and thought she should have been more insistent and not have accepted the doctor saying the tests were expensive, or not reliable anyway, and not to worry—she was very healthy for her age. Most of us trust the words of our doctor and that they must be right, especially since we sometimes see the same primary care physician for decades. We need to be able to trust our doctors, and I'm confident that we generally can. But mostly, we need to trust ourselves, trust our gut. We know ourselves best. If something doesn't feel right, check it out, get a second or third opinion. It may be expensive, though if we ask ourselves, what is the cost of "what if?" or "I should have … "?

THE DREADED BIG C

We all know someone who has won a battle against a cancer. We also all know someone who hasn't.

Cancer isn't choosy; it picks its victims regardless of age, race, sex, gender, and socioeconomic status. Even Steve Jobs, the man who created a veritable tech empire and had access to the best healthcare in the world, died of pancreatic cancer, proving that no amount of money or power can turn back time.

Like many of the diseases we've discussed in this book, there are varying theories about what causes cancer. Research has found a connection between some cancers and what happens in the oral cavity.

In 2015, a group of Korean scientists set out to study periodontitis, the most common chronic inflammatory condition in the mouth.[16] They investigated *Porphyromonas (P.) gingivalis*, a major pathogen of chronic periodontitis, exploring the role it plays in oral cancer.

The results of their study were exciting—and revolutionary. The researchers found that *P. gingivalis* can indeed increase the aggressiveness of oral cancer cells. When it comes to cancer of the mouth, periodontitis poses a serious bacterial risk.

Oral cancer isn't the only kind of cancer that is being studied by researchers as they continue to investigate the importance of a healthy mouth. Scientists have also proposed a link between oral health and esophageal, pancreatic, and colorectal cancer.

Colon cancer is cancer of the large intestine, the lower part of your digestive system; rectal cancer is cancer of the last several inches of the colon. Together, they are referred to as colorectal. Most cases begin as small, noncancerous (benign) clumps of cells called adenomatous polyps; in certain cases, some of these polyps become cancer over time.

About 140,000 people in the US are diagnosed with colorectal cancer each year, and of those, 51,300 are predicted to die from the disease.[17] It is the third most commonly diagnosed cancer and the second leading cause of cancer death.[18]

---

16   N. H. Ha, B. H. Woo, D. J. Kim, *Tumor Biol.* 36 (2015): 9,947. https://doi.org/10.1007/s13277-015-3764-9.

17   "Deaths from Colorectal Cancer," *American Cancer Society*, accessed November 23, 2019, https://www.cancer.org/cancer/colon-rectal-cancer/about/key-statistics.html.

18   "Statistics and Risk Factors," *Colorectal Cancer Alliance*, accessed November 23, 2019, https://www.ccalliance.org/colorectal-cancer-information/statistics-risk-factors.

Two independent studies were recently published in the journal *Cell Host & Microbe*, one from Harvard and the other from Case Western Reserve University. In each study, scientists looked at a strain of mouth bacteria that causes gum disease to determine the role it played in colorectal cancer. The bacteria in question was Fusobacteria.

Fusobacteria start off in the mouth and are frequently associated with gum disease. Earlier studies hadn't observed the bacteria within the actual tumors, which led researchers at Harvard to look at earlier stages of colon cancer to see if this discrepancy was merely an issue of timing.

Their hunch was correct; they found fresh evidence that Fusobacteria were intimately nestled within tumors of the colon. In other words, the bacteria from the oral cavity made their way to the colon, though researchers have not yet definitively proven if the bacteria move through the blood or the gastrointestinal tract.

They didn't stop there. The Harvard researchers found that Fusobacteria elevated the generation of tumors in a mutant mouse strain prone to developing intestinal cancer. Infection with these microbes attracts a particular brand of immune cell—myeloid cells—which the researchers found stimulates the inflammatory responses that can cause cancer.

Inflammation was on the prowl again, this time leading to colorectal cancer. The proof was in the colon.

BREATHE IN, BREATHE OUT

In this chapter we've talked about cancer, but there's another deadly disease that has been linked to oral health (or the lack thereof): lung disease.

Lung disease is another one of those umbrella terms with many diseases nested under it. It is technically any problem in the lungs that prevents them from working properly. Tens of millions of people suffer from lung disease in the US alone.

There are three main types of lung disease:

1. **Airway diseases:** These affect the tubes (airways) that carry oxygen and other gases into and out of the lungs.

2. **Lung-tissue diseases:** These affect the structure of the lung tissue.

3. **Lung-circulation diseases:** These affect the blood vessels in the lungs.

Many lung diseases involve a combination of these three types. Take, for example, COPD, one of the most common lung diseases. COPD comes in two main forms: chronic bronchitis, which involves a long-term cough with mucus, and emphysema, which involves damage to the lungs over time. Smoking, genetics, and infections—including periodontal infections—are responsible for most lung diseases.

There is a fair amount of evidence linking pneumonia to oral health. Scientists have also done a good deal of research to show that good oral hygiene and frequent professional oral healthcare reduce the progression or occurrence of respiratory diseases among high-risk elderly people living in nursing homes, especially those in intensive care units.

Similar studies have shown that lung function decreases with increasing periodontal attachment loss. In layman's terms, your lungs get worse the more the periodontal support around a tooth—the bone and tissue—has been destroyed.

All of this research lends credence to a potential association between periodontitis and chronic pulmonary diseases like COPD.

AND THAT'S NOT ALL

In this chapter we've barely scratched the surface of the different diseases in the body that have been linked to oral health. Additional studies have pointed to a link between inflammation and kidney disease, liver disease, and numerous others.

When I see patients in my practice, these are the kinds of things I'm looking for. I often try to think of ways to help save my patients from these diseases and others. And I know that one way is to focus on prevention.

WHAT CAN YOU DO ABOUT IT?

As with all the diseases we've discussed in this book, there's no tried-and-true method to prevention. You can control and maintain your oral health and other aspects of your lifestyle, but of course there are some things you can't control, like your genetics.

Here's the thing: you *can* control inflammation, starting right in the dentist's chair. You *can* do everything in your power to prevent the inflammation that has been linked to cardiovascular disease; stroke; dementia and Alzheimer's; colorectal, pancreatic, and esophageal cancer; and diseases of the lungs, kidney, and liver.

Yes, additional research is needed. That's how science works. Study by study, case by case, the tide begins to turn. But the writing is on the wall. In the field of oral-systemic health, the body of evidence continues to grow. No one disputes the destructive nature of chronic inflammation. If there is anything you can do to prevent, treat, and correct it, do it. *Do it now.*

The following are some resources that might be helpful:

- http://www.cancer.org
- http://www.emedicinehealth.com
- http://www.webmd.com
- http://www.medicaldaily.com
- http://www.mayoclinic.com
- http://www.webmd.com/lung/lung-diseases-overview

WHAT'S NEXT?

We've talked about a number of diseases that may be caused by the inflammation triggered by periodontal disease. Now we're going to change it up a bit and talk about some *root causes* of inflammation outside the mouth—including obesity, diabetes, and a condition that strikes while you're sound asleep.

That's right: the root causes of disease don't rest, even when you're trying to.

Let's talk about sleep apnea and its stealthy assault.

CHAPTER 7

THE POWER OF A GOOD NIGHT'S SLEEP

People often think that snoring is a sign that someone is sleeping peacefully. In fact, the opposite is true.

I have snored my entire life. I used to think it was normal to snore because my father snored and was a mouth breather. As I gained weight, my snoring worsened—it was so bad that sometimes it would wake me up multiple times a night. It often woke up my wife, and sometimes she made me move to another room.

It was also common for me to wake up in the middle of the night and go to the bathroom, and I was always fatigued—even when I thought I had slept well or for more than eight hours the night before. After work, I often became a zombie on the couch at home, and I rarely had the energy to play with my kids. One Friday, my wife took me to a Taylor Swift concert after work, and I even fell asleep at the concert!

At the time, I thought I was just overworked—I had a busy practice and three young children, so I thought that being tired all the time was normal.

Then, I started learning about airway and how nasal breathing is key to healthier living. I started using nasal dilators and mouth tape to train myself to become a nasal breather instead of a mouth breather. At first, it was tough. Sometimes, I took the nasal dilators out and ripped off the tape while I was sleeping. I would wake up with a dry mouth and still be tired, so I knew I was still breathing through my mouth. But after I got used to them, my wife reported that my snoring decreased. At the same time, I also began to lose weight, which helped improve my airway by reducing obstructions in my throat, and I was waking up with more energy.

For months, I had to wear only the nasal dilators, and I would actually wake up before my alarm almost every morning and feel refreshed. I no longer had the energy crashes during the day, and when I got home, I still had great energy to play with my kids, but I knew I still had other obstructions that needed to be addressed to fully help me with my airway issues. Did I really want to sleep with plastic dilators being shoved up my nose and tape on my mouth every night for the rest of my life?

In 2019, I had nasal surgery to repair my deviated septum and also turbinate reduction to help increase my nasal airflow. The first week was rough because I had stents in my nose and had to breathe through my mouth. I was fatigued every day even though I took the week off from work. I was taking naps throughout the day and realized the detriments that mouth breathing was having on my body

A week later, I had the stents removed from my nose, and the first breath I took was absolutely amazing. I never knew what it felt like to be able to take in that much oxygen! I went to bed, and although I normally set my alarm for 5:30 a.m., I woke up at 4 a.m. and was fully energized! Unfortunately, my gym doesn't open until 5 a.m., so I used the time to catch up on some paperwork I let pile up during my recovery week off. Since then, I consistently wake up before my alarm, I feel refreshed every day, and I have even noticed that my recovery from my workouts is much improved.

More needs to be done to completely eliminate my disrupted sleep—tongue-tie release and myofunctional therapy—but I am living proof that airway matters and am excited to continue my journey to better health.

Most people think that snoring and airway issues predominantly affect the overweight male population, but we know that is not true. In fact, many "young, fit females," like my wife, suffer from airway issues. Still, it's rare that patients come in and tell us that he or she snores. Usually their spouses or significant others are the ones to complain. Many men and women are in denial when faced with the questions of whether they snore or mouth breathe. I've had both male and female patients complain about being too tired or waking up with headaches—with no clue they might be dealing with an airway problem. They think it's normal or stress related.

Most of the time, they don't even know what an airway problem is.

I want to introduce you to Dr. Michael Gelb, a dentist, author, speaker, and sleep specialist at the Gelb Center in New York City. Dr. Gelb specializes in treating temporomandibular joint disorder (TMJ), headaches, sleep disorders, and sleep apnea. He believes that 50 percent of the patients we dentists see in our practice on any given day may struggle with an undiagnosed airway problem. Not a sleep problem. Not a breathing problem. They have a narrowed airway— and they're paying a high price.

Over the years, Dr. Gelb has developed razor-sharp sensibilities. Within a few minutes of examining a patient and listening to them describe their symptoms, he can often tell whether they have an airway problem. It's why he launched the Gelb Center, which now maintains two offices dedicated to AirwayCentric® dentistry, oral-systemic wellness, and anti-inflammatory dentistry. Through his work, he has been able to transform countless lives and has developed the AirwayCentric® Guide (ACG) System for dentists and healthcare providers who wish to implement AirwayCentric® and Complete Health® Practice. More on that later.

In this chapter, I want to share some of Dr. Gelb's wisdom with you. He believes that a clear, healthy, unobstructed airway is the hidden path to well-being—and so do I.

WHAT IS SLEEP APNEA?

Many of us are tired. Day in and day out, we go through our lives in a state of chronic exhaustion. We may go to bed late and get up early. We may have to be up before our kids every morning—we frantically get them ready for school at the same time we get ourselves ready for work. As a consequence of our over-scheduled, overcommitted lives, no one's getting enough sleep.

> Not sleeping well isn't just a minor inconvenience. It can have serious, long-term effects on your health.

We all know that when we are tired, we're not our best self. We're more susceptible to catching a cold or—heaven forbid—being laid flat on our back with a case of the flu.

But not sleeping well isn't just a minor inconvenience. It can have serious, long-term effects on your health.

If you sleep three to four hours a night, you're going to be tired no matter what I do for you. Many of my patients dutifully get their seven to eight hours of sleep a night and still wake up heavy with fatigue. They can't figure out *why* they're so tired, and as we start to trace their symptoms back to the source, we realize something else is going on.

When you breathe, air travels down your throat through your windpipe. The narrowest part of that pathway is in the back of your throat. When you're awake, muscles keep that pathway relatively wide open. When you sleep, those muscles relax, allowing the opening to narrow. The air passing through this narrowed opening may create vibrations. These vibrations in your throat cause snoring.

Snoring is not necessarily indicative of a health issue. But for some people, the throat closes too much, and not enough air can get through to the lungs. When this happens, the brain sends an alarm to open the airway—and you are briefly roused from sleep. Often, this wakes the person sleeping next to you too.

The brain quickly reactivates the muscles that hold the throat open so air can get through again, and once all is free and clear, the brain goes back to sleep. The person lying next to you may remain awake much longer.

This disorder is called obstructive sleep apnea (OSA).

OSA is breathing interrupted by a physical block to airflow despite respiratory effort. Eighty-four percent of sleep apnea is OSA, making it the most common form. The other type of apnea, central sleep apnea (CSA), is breathing interrupted by a *lack* of respiratory effort. Complex or mixed sleep apnea is a combination of OSA and CSA.

All types of sleep apnea create abnormal pauses in breathing— or instances of abnormally low breathing—during sleep. Each pause can last from a few seconds up to whole minutes and may occur five to thirty times (or more) an hour.

Have you ever tried to watch a movie at home, but you keep getting interrupted? Maybe your child keeps running in to ask you questions, or your internet service keeps dropping, or a colleague is bombarding you with text messages, or your dog keeps barking at people walking outside.

If you have to pause your movie five to thirty times in an hour, do you think you'll be able to hold onto the thread of the plot? I'm guessing not!

That's how it is when you have sleep apnea. Your body loses the thread of the plot—the plot being a restful night's sleep.

Symptoms of both OSA and CSA include daytime sleepiness and fatigue, snoring, restless sleep, and awakening with dry mouth or sore throat. One in four patients with OSA suffer from nighttime teeth grinding, which can wear down the teeth and destroy the enamel.

It gets worse. Researchers have revealed that people with OSA show tissue loss in brain regions that help store memory, linking OSA with memory loss. Sleep fragmentation leads to inflammation—and as we've established, inflammation can make you sick.

Despite the long list of symptoms, people who suffer from sleep apnea are rarely aware of having difficulty breathing, even upon waking. You might experience chipped teeth or reflux—little hints and clues leading to sleep apnea—but the disorder is usually recognized only by a partner or friend who has witnessed an episode. Like so many harmful diseases, you may have no idea you're sick. Sleep apnea robs you of your health and vitality—and like a midnight thief, it does it while you sleep.

So far in this book, we've talked about how inflammation is a key player—the central villain, you might say—in oral-systemic health. We've seen how it can drive cardiovascular disease, dementia, and cancer, and we know that bacteria in the gums and mouth can trigger an inflammatory cascade.

Dr. Gelb believes that airway and sleep disorders are the most prominent cause of systemic inflammation, as well as oxidative stress, endothelial dysfunction, and sympathetic overload. This is why he has dedicated his life's work to helping patients open their airways. If he can increase oxygenation to allow deep sleep, he can improve cardiovascular disease, cerebrovascular disease, diabetes, and even dementia and Alzheimer's disease. Oxygen can also help eradicate the microorganisms that exist in the mouth.

Dr. Gelb refers to those microorganisms as "bad bugs." "It is not by coincidence that the bad bugs in our mouth are anaerobic," he says, "meaning they thrive in low-oxygen environments."

What that means is when we open the airway and increase systemic oxygen, it helps to reduce oral bacteria from the inside out, lowering inflammation and reversing chronic disease and dementia.

DON'T LET THE BAD BUGS BITE

We often think of sleep apnea as a disorder that afflicts adults, particularly those who are older and overweight.

It's true that people with low muscle tone and soft tissue around the airway are at a heightened risk for OSA. Common indicators include obesity, BMI greater than thirty, large neck (sixteen inches for women, seventeen inches for men), enlarged tonsils, a large tongue, morning headaches, irritability, mood swings, depression, learning and memory difficulties, and sexual dysfunction. Risk of OSA rises with increase in body weight, active smoking, and age. Diabetics or borderline diabetics are up to three times more likely to have it.

Opportunities for prevention are available far earlier than we might think. By age three or four, kids can already be dealing with allergies that negatively affect their breathing or other factors that make them mouth breathers. They might snore, which we think is cute.

But it's not cute. For kids, having even one event an hour, one moment when their sleep is interrupted, can have a devastating effect. Interrupted sleep can affect the normal development of the prefrontal cortex, and then suddenly your child might get diagnosed as ADHD or other disorders, which might have been prevented by ensuring uninterrupted, healthful sleep.

If, on the other hand, the prefrontal cortex develops the way it's supposed to, it yields positive neurobehavioral and neurocognitive results. This will affect the hippocampus, the brain center of emotion, memory, and the autonomic nervous system. A healthy prefrontal cortex can make your children far less susceptible to dementia and cognitive impairment later in life. It can even decrease the risk of anxiety and depression.

You wouldn't believe how many patients come to my practice with anxiety—and since many of them see me more often than their general practitioner, I'm the one they talk to about it. Dr. Gelb has gotten incredible results with his patients when it comes to anxiety. "I can get rid of anxiety by 50 percent within two weeks," he says, "just by taking the airway that's being pinched and opening it up."

If you're anxious or depressed, you should always speak to a psychologist or psychiatrist. That said, I'm encouraged by the work doctors like Dr. Gelb are doing. Unblocking the airway could be another important tool in your tool kit when it comes to combating mental illness, including drug-resistant anxiety and depression.

Good sleep habits and preventive measures can make a crucial difference to the well-being of your children, both now and in the future. Sleep is when the brain recharges. Human growth hormone gets released at night, which is pivotal as your child grows and develops.

> Unblocking the airway could be another important tool in your tool kit when it comes to combating mental illness, including drug-resistant anxiety and depression.

I believe you can prevent your kids from ever getting sleep apnea. And since men are more likely to suffer from sleep apnea than women at a three-to-one ratio, just think of the positive effect this will have on your child's future relationships. Your sons will never become snorers like me, and your daughters will never become like my wife, married to a man she has to exile to the guest room just to get a good night's sleep!

WHAT CAN YOU DO ABOUT IT?

The current and developing research on sleep apnea is very hopeful. Treatment of OSA with continuous positive airway pressure (CPAP) and oral devices—more on those in a moment—improves levels of inflammatory markers. This is significant, considering atherosclerosis (the disease of the arteries we discussed in chapter 4) is an inflammatory disease. OSA may be the link between atherosclerosis and periodontal disease that the dental community has been so interested in, since the association between these two conditions has been supported by evidence-based research.

Dr. Gelb has enjoyed phenomenal success in his practice. He and his team have developed a personalized treatment plan involving treatment of periodontal disease, laser periodontal therapy, and tray delivery system. This customized oral-hygiene plan also helps disrupt the colonization of bacteria and expose the hiding places of the bad bugs. Dr. Gelb's team of sleep experts monitors blood markers for inflammation, keeping track of how well they are doing to bring systemic inflammation down to ideal levels to keep patients at their healthiest.

At the heart of Dr. Gelb's work is the ACG™ AirwayCentric® System: the first fully integrated day and night oral appliance approach to solving airway issues by integrating Airway and Sleep with TMJ. The system includes six appliances that complement the traditional ProSomnus [IA] Platform, including the day and the night appliances.

These appliances stop the lower jaw from dropping back at night, preventing a collapse of the airway during sleep. The main focus of the night appliances is to alleviate OSA and snoring and to improve oxygenation, promoting more restorative sleep.

These are not your average oral appliances. They won't close the airway and can alleviate clicking and locking, headaches, and neck pain. You may awaken more refreshed and with better focus and memory. And of course, there are the huge, long-term benefits in preventing cardiovascular disease and dementia.

Alleviating the symptoms of sleep apnea may mean more than wearing an appliance. For many patients, it may also mean orthodontics, removal of tonsils and adenoids, tongue-tie release and myofunctional therapy, and maybe even jaw surgery. The goal of wearing an appliance, which for some people is combined with CPAP, is to help the person get more oxygen and better sleep. However, the ideal situation is to be able to get a great night's sleep without such devices, and that involves a team approach and treatment that can take years. The appliance gets you to a place where you are comfortable and can breathe. The team can then get you into that position so you can breathe on your own.

At the end of the day, what if all we really need is a good night's sleep?

The following are some resources that might be helpful:

- https://www.drmichaelgelb.com/nightguard-2-0/
- https://www.drmichaelgelb.com/acg-system/
- http://www.sleepfoundation.org
- http://www.mayoclinic.com
- http://www.chestnet.org
- http://www.perioimplantadvisory.com

WHAT'S NEXT?

In the next chapter, we will discuss a condition in which a little extra weight is not only normal—it's exactly what you want. You'll also learn about how obesity and diabetes can be complicating factors for disease by aiding and abetting inflammation in the body.

If you want to know how periodontal disease can lead to pregnancy complications and preterm birth, read on.

CHAPTER 8

BABIES, BELLIES, AND BLOOD SUGAR

Dr. Lorna Okada, a friend and referring dentist, generously shared the following story with me about her challenges in having children.

My greatest fear when I was in my twenties was whether I would be able to have children. It wasn't a fear that I would obsess over, just something that would linger in the back of my head and would surface whenever I would contemplate what the future held. So naturally for me, every time I would get into a serious relationship, I would think about whether this was someone I would want to have kids with.

Darrell and I got married the year before my thirtieth birthday. I could've said that I was twenty-nine, but ever since I had gone for my yearly OB-GYN appointment the year before and was told that women who had children before they were thirty were less likely to have breast cancer, that statistic (which I never verified to be true or not) added to my hypochondriac mind. We got pregnant pretty quickly after we started trying and were lucky to have an easy and healthy pregnancy. Connor was born and brought a lot of fulfillment and joy to our busy lives.

Next thing we knew, Connor had turned three, we were pretty well adjusted to family life and trying our best to juggle being full-time working parents, and we started to try for baby number two. Months of excitement and anticipation led to disappointment and frustration from not conceiving. We had sensitive discussions about whether to pursue fertility help or just be happy with our family of three. After three consultations, failed intrauterine insemination, multiple acupuncture appointments, and Darrell going through a procedure himself, over the course of two years, I finally decided to pull the trigger on going through in vitro fertilization (IVF). This was something I needed to do for myself so I could find closure to my nagging monthly moment of depression when I would start my period. I needed to take action because the advice, "Just stop thinking or worrying about it, and then it will happen," wasn't helping.

Couples who haven't experienced issues with fertility have the luxury of not having gone through the emotional roller coaster that can drag on for months and then years. This anxiety and tension played a major role in my well-being at the time. I was desperate to make some changes—anything that was going to make a difference. Diet, exercise, any extra supplements or treatments—I looked into them all. Another major factor was cost—the IVF process wasn't covered by our insurance, and the medications were only partially covered.

There are different tiers to the price of treatment, depending on the customized treatment plan. And to no surprise, I needed almost every extra procedure there was, and it cost more because I was overweight. Darrell joked that this process was his new car driving away. This was only partially funny, because the IVF clinic I had decided on was a good thirty- to forty-minute drive with no traffic, and of course most of my appointments were during the morning commute.

Once I had decided on the IVF clinic, I was all in on what was recommended. There were strict guidelines on diet and weight; I tried my best. It was a difficult journey, and I had to make a lot of changes on top of the regimen of injections and medications. Being a mom with a busy practice didn't make going to last-minute appointments that my body dictated easy. Going to multiple appointments over the course of several months was trying, including the multiple blood draws, IVs for infusions, IV sedation for the egg retrieval, and then the embryo transfer. My buttocks would hurt so bad from the oil-based hormones that needed to get injected in the same two-inch area day after day. I started making friends with the pharmacist at the specialty pharmacy where I would pick up all my meds.

Unexpected bills brought extra financial stress that made things harder. I can see how they can't tell you all the possible costs involved, but it wasn't easy having to make a choice to spend thousands of extra dollars to genetically test the embryos, an option the doctor recommended but said wasn't necessary.

I kept telling myself that we were going to give it our all, but if it didn't work out, at least we had our one child.

I didn't want to get my hopes too high, for I feared the depression that might hit if things didn't work out. Connor and my family and friends were the strong support system I needed to stay positive and enthusiastic.

I'm happy to say that everything worked out—I had an easy pregnancy, healthy birth, and quick recovery. We have our beautiful, confident, and independent daughter, Savannah, and feel so blessed and grateful, never looking back.

There are other stories that don't end so happily. Women who do not maintain a healthy mouth during pregnancy can suffer severe and heartbreaking consequences. Though the science is still evolving, studies have suggested a link between inflammation and pregnancy complications such as preterm labor, preeclampsia (rise in blood pressure), and even stillbirth.

This is not something any pregnant couple should have to endure—which is why we need to talk about it, to ensure it never happens to you.

BACTERIA IS BAD FOR YOUR BABY

Here's a statistic that may surprise you: according to the World Health Organization, the US ranks sixth among the top ten countries for premature births.[19] Twelve percent—more than one in nine of all births—are preterm. That's half a million babies each year.

Dr. Yiping Han is a researcher at the College of Dental Medicine at Columbia University. Her focus is on oral microbiology; she

---

19   Partnership for Maternal, Newborn, and Child Health, *Born Too Soon: The Global Action Report on Preterm Birth*, accessed July 5, 2019, http://www.who.int/pmnch/media/news/2012/preterm_birth_report/en/index3.html.

studies how oral bacteria cause infections in the mouth and elsewhere in the body.

In 1996, a study was published providing the first evidence that women with periodontitis had a tendency to deliver premature and low-birth-weight babies. Since then, there have been a number of supporting epidemiological studies. In a paper published in the *Journal of Dental Research*, Dr. Han dug deep into the existing research. She concluded that "evidence is accumulating that oral bacteria may translocate directly into the pregnant uterus, causing localized inflammation and adverse pregnancy outcomes."[20]

In layman's terms, this means that if bacteria from the mouth sneak into the bloodstream, they spread everywhere. Sound familiar? Some make their way into the uterus, where they can lead to infection, causing the sack of fluid to break prematurely, preterm labor, and— in worst-case scenarios—stillbirth.

To put it bluntly, it could kill the baby.

The findings from Dr. Han's studies are significant because they challenge the existing paradigm in the medical community. When doctors find an intrauterine infection, it's usually believed to originate in the vaginal tract. But Dr. Han's studies show that the bacteria may *not* come from the vaginal tract—and could very well come from the mouth through the bloodstream. In fact, oral bacteria might account for anywhere between 10 and 30 percent of these infections.

Needless to say, the cost of bacteria invading a pregnant woman's uterus is incredibly high—physically, financially, and emotionally. When a family loses a baby, it can be crushing. Grieving parents often wonder, "Was this my fault? What did I do wrong?" It breaks

---

20 Yiping Han, "Oral Health and Adverse Pregnancy Outcomes—What's Next?" *J. Dental Research* 90, no. 3 (March 2011): 289–93 https://www.ncbi.nlm.nih.gov/pubmed/21041548.

my heart to hear that question. I would love to prevent this kind of loss for as many parents as possible. It's a mission I strongly believe in—and one of the reasons I wanted to write this book.

This infection can also infect the uterus in women not yet pregnant. It can make it exceedingly difficult to conceive in the first place or kill the baby before it's even a known pregnancy; most miscarriages happen in the first twelve weeks.[21]

Compounding the problem in some, there is strong science to support the thesis that women on fertility treatments may have trouble getting pregnant because the extra hormones given to stimulate fertility are absorbed into the estrogen receptors in their gums. If there is already bacterial infection present, the hormones can exacerbate it.

Intuitively, the oral-systemic connection makes sense. An infected uterus is a high-risk place for a tiny human to develop. A healthy mouth contributes to an environment that can allow for a healthy, successful pregnancy.

WHAT CAN YOU DO ABOUT IT?

We've all heard about strange pregnancy cravings, whether we've had them ourselves, known women who have them, or seen them on TV. We joke about a mom-to-be needing her sardines and ice cream, but at the end of the day, she would do well to ditch the ice cream. The more frequently you give in to the craving for sugary snacks, the greater the chance of developing tooth decay. Studies have shown that the bacteria responsible for tooth decay pass from the mother to the child in utero. Not something you want your baby to inherit!

---

21 "What Is a Miscarriage?" *WebMD*, accessed July 5, 2019, https://www.webmd.com/baby/understanding-miscarriage-basics#1.

There are other aspects of pregnancy that make it more difficult to maintain good oral hygiene. For example, pregnant women with acid reflux are at a greater risk of tooth erosion and periodontal problems, as the acid begins to thin and wear

> If you are experiencing acid reflux, you should talk to your dentist about ways of combating these negative effects.

away the enamel—the protective coating of the teeth—leaving them weakened. If you are experiencing acid reflux, you should talk to your dentist about ways of combating these negative effects. Many times, acid reflux and/or gastroesophageal reflux disease are related to airway issues.

Increasingly, insurance companies are recognizing the value of healthy gums during pregnancy and are encouraging hygiene cleanings—and so do I.

Now let's talk about when you're carrying extra weight that's *not* a bun in the oven.

OBESITY, DIABETES, AND PERIODONTAL DISEASE: A VICIOUS CYCLE

We've touched briefly on obesity and diabetes as complicating factors of other diseases, but I wanted to add a few words here. Obesity is a medical condition in which excess body fat has accumulated to the extent that it may have an adverse effect on health. More than one-third of US adults are obese. It is well known that obesity can increase the likelihood of sleep apnea, heart disease, type 2 diabetes, and certain types of cancer.

In a study published in the *Journal of Periodontology*, obese individuals between the ages of eighteen and thirty-four were found to have a rate of periodontal disease *76 percent higher* than individuals within a healthy weight.[22] Obese patients have more tooth decay and more missing teeth. Since diet is partly to blame, I always encourage my obese patients to avoid sugary drinks, limit snacking, and eat a well-balanced diet. Bacteria love sugar as much as the rest of us, and when they feed on the sugars in food, they make acids. Over time, these acids destroy enamel, resulting in tooth decay.

Obesity and diabetes are often linked, insofar as obese men and women—especially those with belly fat—are at a higher risk for type 2 diabetes. And to further connect the dots, gum disease is considered the sixth complication of diabetes. Patients with uncontrolled type 2 diabetes are at a much higher risk for gum disease.

It's a vicious cycle because severe periodontal disease can increase blood sugar—and poor sugar control is what causes diabetes. Diabetes is a condition in which a person has high blood sugar (glucose). This occurs either because the insulin production is inadequate, because the body's cells do not respond to insulin, or both.

Insulin's job is to pull glucose out of the blood and give it to tissues that need it. If you have an active periodontal infection, your blood sugar level stays elevated, because when you have an infection of any kind in your body, it stimulates your liver to release sugar in an effort to fight off the infection.

Additionally, studies have shown that diabetics have a decreased ability to fight infections, including infection in the gums. This increases the bacterial load in the mouth, making gum inflamma-

---

22   M. S. Al–Zahrani, N. F. Bissada, and E. A. Borawskit, "Obesity and Periodontal Disease in Young, Middle Aged and Older Adults," *J Periodontol* 74 (2003): 610–615.

tion worse. Together, these increase the likelihood that bacteria enter the bloodstream to drive disease at distant sites. We've all heard the nightmare stories of diabetics who have had to amputate toes or even limbs. Don't let this happen to you—understanding the oral-systemic connection can make all the difference.

Just look at Donatella. She found out she had diabetes because of failed implants. She had been referred to me and needed three implants in her upper jaw along with some bone grafting. She was overweight and had high blood pressure and had not been to the doctor recently for a medical exam. She presented with all the signs of metabolic syndrome, but it was very early in my career at the time—I was just getting started—and I did not delve deeper. Back then, I did not understand the oral-systemic connection like I do now. All I knew was that she wanted implants, and I was eager to place them for her.

After the surgery, she developed infections, which ended up causing both the implants and bone grafts to fail. After a second bone graft failed, I talked to her about getting a blood test and medical exam. She was all for it as she did not want to go through any more surgery.

Her HbA1c (blood sugar) levels were through the roof—she was an uncontrolled diabetic. No wonder she was having trouble healing. I told her that I would see her again after she was cleared for surgery by her medical doctor.

A year later, she came in wanting to have the implants and grafting done again, and I had to do a double take as I did not even recognize her! She had lost more than fifty pounds and looked like a different person. Plus, her blood sugar levels were finally under control.

She thanked me for saving her life.

This time, her bone grafts and implants succeeded. She had more than a new smile; she had a new lease on life. What was the worst failure of my early career became one of my biggest successes, not just because we gave her great implants, but because we helped her turn her life around. She was not only healthier; she was more confident and just completely transformed.

By now you probably see the circular nature of these conditions: diabetes can lead to periodontal disease, and periodontal disease can cause—and exacerbate—diabetes, and these are then in turn related to other diseases like Alzheimer's disease and cardiovascular disease.

Researchers recently performed a study premised on the question, "Which comes first, diabetes or periodontal disease?"

They followed the test subjects for years. One in particular stood out, a happy, healthy thirty-five-year-old woman with neither periodontal disease nor diabetes when the study began. About three-and-a-half years later, she developed severe periodontal disease. So much bone was lost that her teeth actually migrated, and some of her back teeth were at risk of falling out.

What the researchers found was that, in the time between the two visits, this woman had also developed diabetes. If a patient has diabetes and also has periodontal disease, the periodontal disease makes diabetes worse—and vice versa.

This is a perfect example of the interaction between the mouth and the body. The oral-systemic link can work in *both* directions, a deleterious dance of cause and effect.

The following are some resources that might be helpful regarding pregnancy:

- http://www.americanpregnancy.org
- http://www.webmd.com/oral-health/dental-care-pregnancy
- http://www.disabled-world.com
- http://www.whattoexpect.com
- http://dentalhealthandwellnessboston.com
- https://www.perio.org/consumer

The following are some resources that might be helpful regarding obesity and diabetes:

- http://www.obesityaction.org
- http://www.cdc.gov/obesity/data/adult.html
- http://www.medicalnewstoday.com/info/diabetes
- https://www.perio.org/consumer/gum-disease-and-diabetes.htm

WHAT'S NEXT?

We've talked about the relationship between inflammation and cardiovascular disease, dementia, cancers, sleep apnea, pregnancy complications, obesity, and diabetes.

We've talked about the vast and far-reaching consequences of periodontal disease on your health, happiness, and life.

But what are the broader implications of the oral-systemic link? As we move into a third era of healthcare, how do our choices affect our cities, our country, and our world?

CHAPTER 9

THE COST OF DOING NOTHING IS TOO GREAT

I'm proud to be an American. I think we live in the greatest country in the world.

But to be honest with you, I believe we have some work to do when it comes to keeping people healthy, happy, and free to live long, independent lives. Our current healthcare system isn't about "health" at all—and that needs to change. We have a *sick care* system.

Today's medical costs can be crushing. They certainly aren't competitive with other countries: healthcare in the United States is *twice* as expensive as in Europe and four times as expensive as in Mexico, Japan, India, and China. Major companies have figured this out, which is why they've created incentive programs and wellness initiatives to encourage preventive care.

Our country has hit a pivotal inflection point. Healthcare has to become less expensive, and in my mind, the only way to accomplish that is to better maintain good health and focus on prevention and inflammation—and that starts with taking better care of our mouths.

In 2014, a landmark paper was published in the *American Journal of Preventive Medicine*.[23] In the study—the first of its kind—researchers from the University of Pennsylvania conducted a comprehensive, five-year project in which they evaluated the claims of nearly 1.7 million patients covered by Highmark Health and United Concordia Dental. The researchers were looking specifically at patients with chronic medical conditions and also pregnant women.

What they discovered was remarkable. Out of almost 1.7 million patients, 338,891 people who suffered from a chronic medical condition had also been diagnosed with periodontal disease. That's a solid 20 percent.

The researchers didn't stop there. They drilled down into the dollars and cents of the research, lasering in on patients who were actually *treated* for their gum disease. They found the annual financial savings to be impressive. People with coronary artery disease saved on average $1,090 yearly on their annual medical costs. Diabetics saved an average of $2,840 yearly. People who had suffered from a stroke saved a whopping $5,681. Women who were pregnant saved $2,433.

In my opinion, the savings in this study was significantly underestimated. The Centers for Disease Control and Prevention estimates that 47.2 percent—nearly *half of American adults*—have periodontal disease.[24] The fact that only 20 percent of the study participants had periodontal disease noted in their dental records proves the condition

---

23   "The Mouth: The Missing Piece to Overall Wellness and Lower Medical Costs," United Concordia, accessed July 5, 2019, https://www.unitedconcordia.com/docs/united%20concordia%20oral%20health%20whitepaper.pdf.

24   P. I. Eke, B. A. Dye, L. Wei, G. O. Thornton-Evans, and R. J. Genco, "Prevalence of Periodontitis in Adults in the United States: 2009 and 2010," *J. Dental Research* 91, no. 10 (2012): 914–920, http://journals.sagepub.com/doi/abs/10.1177/0022034512457373.

is severely underdiagnosed. If all those with periodontal disease had been identified and treated, the savings would have been much, much higher.

Thousands of dollars saved, simply by getting a healthier mouth.

PROUD TO HAVE A HEALTHY MOUTH

If the mouth is the gateway to complete health, then it follows that keeping our mouths healthy is the gateway to a stronger, healthier America.

But change doesn't happen on its own. There is a specially trained group of men and women in this country who will have to step forward and offer preventive care if we want to kick-start the revolution.

I'm one of them. Your periodontist.

Or if you prefer something a little fancier, "oral-systemic specialist."

I'm guessing that, before you read this book, dentists would *not* have been the first professionals to come to mind when you imagined solving our nation's health problems. But if you think about it, we dentists are in the *ideal* position to make a tremendous influence on our healthcare system.

Generally, people are already in the habit of visiting the dentist every six months—way more often than the average American visits their primary care physician. And as you now understand better, preventing disease is significantly

> People are already in the habit of visiting the dentist every six months—way more often than the average American visits their primary care physician.

less costly than trying to cure people once they have it. Considering the 162 diseases with early warning signs that can be detected in the mouth, we dentists may in fact be the *perfect* health professional to prevent and reverse disease.

In other words, the system is already set up for the solution.

There has to be a contextual shift in how we think about the mouth. As Dr. Whitney says, we need to move into the third era of dentistry. Many dentists are still trapped in the old-school way of thinking. They subscribe to the "drill, fill, bill" mentality, or like so many physicians today, "treat it and beat it." We're trained to find the chief complaint and fix it. But that's a reactive care dentist. That's not the person who's going to be leading the revolution.

The times we're living in call for a new kind of dentistry—and to go with it, a new kind of dental team.

When we graduated from dental school, we were taught to be problem-solvers. In this new context of complete health, we understand that the body affects the mouth and the mouth affects the body.

For me personally, this shift in mindset has allowed me to look at the whole patient. When I started asking people about their general medical history and their family history, I found that many of them hadn't been to see their physician for a checkup in years. That gave me the opportunity to engage in conversations with them about everything from smoking to exercise to getting an appointment with their primary care physician to get a long-overdue physical.

When a patient comes into my practice, I don't just ask, "Is anything bothering you?" with the intent of fixing it and sending them on their merry way. I look at their health from a wider scope. When I'm treating their periodontal disease, I'm also looking for signs and symptoms of other diseases or conditions. I encourage them to go see their general practitioner to discuss the concerns we raised in the dental office.

I treat the whole person, not just the mouth. My patients see me and my team as more than just a dentist office. We care about their total body health and well-being.

Am I trying to replace physicians? Not at all. I want to *partner* with my fellow medical professionals. If the mouth is the first line of defense, that means I have a lot of responsibility to keep you healthy. I have valuable information about your health that I can share with your primary care physician or other doctors—and I don't take that responsibility lightly. Neither do my hygienists, who are critical to providing the best care we can offer.

We are assuming our needed role in the integrated model of healthcare. When I think of the future of our country as Complete Health Dentistry® takes root, I have a very clear vision. I imagine the full spectrum of healthcare practitioners coming together to provide you with the very best in holistic, integrated care. I imagine physicians understanding and embracing the importance of the oral cavity as a powerful gateway to complete health, not a separate island cut off from the rest of our body.

I imagine a world in which the public government, insurance carriers, physicians, dentists, hygienists, pharmacists, dieticians, and all health professionals understand dentistry as the first line of defense against sickness and debilitating disease.

I imagine patients who are excited to assume ownership of their own health, taking proactive and preventive measures to ensure they live a long, healthy life.

That's the reason our office practices Complete Health Dentistry®. I believe dentists can change the world.

But I can't do it alone. To turn the tide as we move boldly into the third era of healthcare, there's one more person who plays a pivotal role.

You.

CHAPTER 10

THE COMPLETE HEALTH DENTISTRY® TRANSFORMATION

Complete Health Dentistry® has helped me feel that I'm more than "just a dentist." I now feel like an integral part of the healthcare team for patients. My team and I love knowing that we are not just making teeth healthier; we're making people healthier.

These days, we talk to our patients in a different context. No longer are we "selling" dentistry. Take, for example, scaling and root planing, a procedure that can help restore gum health. Before it was, "We need to do a deep cleaning since you have deep pockets in your gums." At that point, patients usually just wanted to know whether the procedure was covered by insurance. Now, a typical explanation is more along the lines of, "As a diabetic, you do not have the same healing abilities as other people because your body is unable to fight the bacteria in your mouth as effectively as a nondiabetic. These bacteria cause active inflammation in your mouth, and the bacteria can go through the ulcerations of your bleeding gums and can get into your bloodstream and cause other diseases and complications. Did you know that periodontal disease, the disease that you have, is linked directly to heart disease and Alzheimer's disease, just to name a few?" At that point, patients are usually more amenable to whatever needs to be done to help them live longer and be healthier.

What we recommend is bacterial and DNA testing. Even though these are not covered by insurance, they can help us see when someone has problems below the surface or when they are genetically predisposed to certain diseases.

In most mild and some moderate forms of periodontal disease, a deep cleaning (scaling and root planing) and more frequent cleanings (every three to four months instead of every six months) are needed. In more severe cases, sometimes gum surgery is necessary. The good news is that today's gum surgery is not the gum surgery your grandma went through years ago.

> Treating gum disease is not a "one and done" but a lifetime of commitment and treatment. I mean, it's your body we are talking about!

We are proud to offer laser gum surgery, or Laser-Assisted New Attachment Procedure (LANAP). This is a minimally invasive gum procedure where we use the power of the laser to kill the bacteria of your mouth and attempt to regenerate the lost bone that the gum disease may have caused. Because this surgery is minimally invasive, most patients go back to work the next day with little to no discomfort! So we are making patients healthier, with less discomfort, and with the ability to regenerate their lost bone in just one sitting.

Once a patient's gum disease is under control, we have to maintain this health for life. Treating gum disease is not a "one and done" but a lifetime of commitment and treatment. I mean, it's your body we are talking about!

Because of this, we offer to all of our patients Perio Protect, trays that allow patients to get at-home protection against oral disease in between dental visits. Daily use of the custom-fabricated trays for just ten to fifteen minutes can get oxygen via hydrogen peroxide gels into the oxygen-free environment below the gum line and kill the bacteria while also whitening teeth, and when we explain this, we find more patients are interested in using them. Just imagine, you only get the bacteria under your gums treated once every six months when you go in for your regular cleanings. Now this can be done every single day while you take a shower or drive to work.

In short, Complete Health Dentistry® is a much more fulfilling way to practice. We love helping patients understand the importance of their oral health and want to do whatever it takes to help them be healthy.

I've had patients cry in my chair over the excitement of knowing that they can be helped. And as they become healthier, they become the practice's best advocates. They tell their family, friends, and coworkers about our practice and how we look at things differently and care about our patients' health. They know that the mouth is connected to a body, and if we can make the mouth healthier, we can also help the body and mind.

"WE SAVED A LIFE TODAY"

Whenever I talk about airway and the oral-systemic connection to patients, family, or friends, I get different reactions. Some people are really excited to hear about it and are motivated to get healthier. Some love the info but are not ready to make the changes needed. And a small percentage just do not care. That used to discourage me, but after my own journey, I realize that it's a lot of information for people to take in. Some just need time to let it sink in, and others need to do their own research before they get it. It's the same reaction I had to my trainer when he told me about intermittent fasting. I had heard about it but was not ready to commit to it at that time. But when I did, I was all in and was ultimately able to reap the benefits. I had to wait for my time to be successful.

> If you are ready to proceed on the journey to better oral and overall health, look for local providers who subscribe to the concept of an oral-systemic connection.

If you are ready to proceed on the journey to better oral and overall health, look for local providers who subscribe to the concept of an oral-systemic connection. That may be a dentist, periodontist, orthodontist, or sleep medicine doctor, who may refer you to another specialist such as an ENT, oral surgeon, or myofunctional therapist. Whatever it takes, there is a network of doctors to help you.

Depending on your specific needs, your journey may be short and resolved fairly easily, or it may take longer and require more aggressive treatment. No matter the solution, it is worth it to help you breathe better, reduce your inflammatory load, and live longer.

The more you know about the oral-systemic connection, the more you share with friends and family, the better chance you have of saving the life of someone you love.

The biggest joy in my practice is being told by my team that "we saved someone's life today." We know that every patient is more than just a mouth that needs attention. You are someone with a family and friends and people who love you. We know that the care we provide affects everyone connected to you.

TAKE ACTION NOW

Now that you've read all about the oral-systemic connection, I encourage you to do the following:

1. Make an appointment with one of the skilled doctors at the Ueno Center, or see a restorative dentist who is well versed in oral-systemic health and airway. A comprehensive treatment plan needs to be made with the proper referrals, and that starts with an initial consultation with the right provider.

2. Educate yourself as much as you can about oral-systemic health and airway. Research online. Buy books on Amazon. Whatever it takes. Then take a look at yourself and your family. Do your parents or siblings have problems with clenching and grinding? Did they have periodontal treatments in the past? Is there Alzheimer's disease, heart disease, cancer, or other disease in your family history?

3. Understand that everyone's journey in oral-systemic health is different, and a custom-made plan will be devised for you. Some of these plans can take years, but the light at the end of the tunnel is a healthier you. Always keep that in mind. Some people can burn out during the course of treatment, but do your best to stay the course. And make sure you are ready to begin in the first place. If you say yes for the sake of saying yes, you will burn out. If you are not ready, take the time you need to get yourself to the point that you are ready. Again, everyone's journey is different.

Want to know more? We have a lot of great info about the oral-systemic connection at www.uenodentalcenter.com. Why not reach out and let us help motivate you to achieve your best health? The doctors and team at the Ueno Center are excited to be a part of your team to bring you to better oral and systemic health so you can live your best life for your friends, family, and yourself.

ABOUT THE AUTHOR

Dr. Jeremy Ueno is a periodontist in Campbell, California, in the heart of Silicon Valley. His practice is focused on dental implants, laser gum surgery, and making his patients healthier through the oral-systemic connection. He received his surgical training at the esteemed Columbia University in New York City. Dr. Ueno also runs the Practi(CE)nter where he teaches advanced continuing education to other dentists to help increase the quality of care of patients in the Bay Area. He lectures both nationally and internationally and is highly respected in his field.

The oral-systemic connection saved Dr. Ueno's life. As he learned more about the connections between the mouth and the body, including airway and sleep apnea, he began to look at himself in the mirror more. He made a change in every aspect of his life, including getting surgery to help him breathe better. He lost over fifty pounds in one year and his health dramatically improved. He definitely believes in practicing what you preach and loves helping his patients and their families live healthier lives.

NOTES

Lester Breslow, "Health Measurement in the Third Era of Health," *Am J Public Health* 96, no. 1 (January 2006): 17–19, https://www.ncbi.nlm.nih.gov/pmc/articles/PMC1470427/.

P. J. Pussinen, P. Jousilahti, G. Alfthan, T. Palosuo, S. Asikainen, and V. Salomaa, "Antibodies to Periodontal Pathogens Are Associated with Coronary Heart Disease," *Arterioscler Thromb Vasc Biol* 23 (2003): 1,250–1,254.

P. J. Pussinen, G. Alfthan, H. Rissanen, A. Reunanen, S. Asikainen, and P. Knekt, "Antibodies to Periodontal Pathogens and Stroke Risk," *Stroke* 35 (2004): 2,020–2,023.

E. V. Kozarov, B. R. Dorn, C. E. Shelburne, W. A. Dunn, and A. Progulske-Fox, "Human Atherosclerotic Plaque Contains Viable Invasive *Actinobacillus actinomycetemcomitans* and *Porphyromonas gingivalis*," *Arteriosclerosis, Thrombosis, and Vascular Biology* 25 (2005): e17–e18.

B. Pihlstrom, J. Hodges, B. Michalowicz, J. C. Wohlfahrt, and R. Garcia, "Promoting Oral Health Care Because of Its Possible Effect on Systemic Disease Is Premature and May Be Misleading," *JADA* 149 (2018): 401–403.

J. Russo, S. Estep, S. Maples, D. Wilkerson, M. Milligan, V. Richards, J. Lazarus et al., "AAOSH Responds to *JADA* Editorial That Claims Promoting Oral-Systemic Connection Is 'Premature and Misleading,'" *American Academy for Oral Systemic Health*, June 15, 2018, https://aaosh.org/jada-response.

Brad Bale and Amy Doneen, "The Vital Importance of the Mouth-Body Connection," *Oral Systemic Link*, accessed

April 20, 2017, http://oralsystemiclink.net/patients/profile/
the-vital-importance-of-the-mouth-body-connection.

"Fact and Figures," Alzheimer's Association, accessed November 23,
2019, https://www.alz.org/alzheimers-dementia/facts-figures.

"Fact and Figures," Alzheimer's Association.

"Facts and Figures," Alzheimer's Association.

"Dementia vs Alzheimer's," Fisher Center for Alzheimer's Research
Foundation, accessed July 5, 2019, http://www.alzinfo.org/
understand-alzheimers/dementia/.

Lauren Ingeno, "Do Infections Cause Alzheimer's Disease?" *Drexel
University News Blog*, accessed July 5, 2019, https://newsblog.drexel.
edu/2016/02/10/do-infections-cause-alzheimers-disease/.

Judith. J. Miklossy, "Alzheimer's Disease – A Neurospirochetosis" *J.
Neuroinflammation* 8, no. 90 (August 2011), https://www.ncbi.nlm.
nih.gov/pubmed/21816039.

H. Allen, "Alzheimer's Disease: A Novel Hypothesis Integrating
Spirochetes, Biofilm, and the Immune System," *J. Neuroinfectious
Diseases* 7, no. 1 (2016), https://www.ncbi.nlm.nih.gov/pmc/articles/
PMC5008232/.

Mark Wheeler, "Memory Loss Associated with Alzheimer's Reversed for First Time," *UCLA Newsroom*, accessed
July 5, 2019, http://newsroom.ucla.edu/releases/
memory-loss-associated-with-alzheimers-reversed-for-first-time.

N. H. Ha, B. H. Woo, D. J. Kim, *Tumor Biol.* 36 (2015): 9,947.
https://doi.org/10.1007/s13277-015-3764-9.

"Deaths from Colorectal Cancer," *American Cancer Society*, accessed November 23, 2019, https://www.cancer.org/cancer/colon-rectal-cancer/about/key-statistics.html.

"Statistics and Risk Factors," *Colorectal Cancer Alliance*, accessed November 23, 2019, https://www.ccalliance.org/colorectal-cancer-information/statistics-risk-factors.

Partnership for Maternal, Newborn, and Child Health, *Born Too Soon: The Global Action Report on Preterm Birth*, accessed July 5, 2019, http://www.who.int/pmnch/media/news/2012/preterm_birth_report/en/index3.html.

Yiping Han, "Oral Health and Adverse Pregnancy Outcomes—What's Next?" *J. Dental Research* 90, no. 3 (March 2011): 289–93 https://www.ncbi.nlm.nih.gov/pubmed/21041548.

"What Is a Miscarriage?" *WebMD*, accessed July 5, 2019, https://www.webmd.com/baby/understanding-miscarriage-basics#1.

M. S. Al–Zahrani, N. F. Bissada, and E. A. Borawskit, "Obesity and Periodontal Disease in Young, Middle Aged and Older Adults," *J Periodontol* 74 (2003): 610–615.

"The Mouth: The Missing Piece to Overall Wellness and Lower Medical Costs," United Concordia, accessed July 5, 2019, https://www.unitedconcordia.com/docs/united%20concordia%20oral%20health%20whitepaper.pdf.

P. I. Eke, B. A. Dye, L. Wei, G. O. Thornton-Evans, and R. J. Genco, "Prevalence of Periodontitis in Adults in the United States: 2009 and 2010," *J. Dental Research* 91, no. 10 (2012): 914–920, http://journals.sagepub.com/doi/abs/10.1177/0022034512457373.